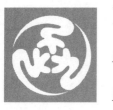

HONEY, MUD,
MAGGOTS, AND OTHER
MEDICAL MARVELS

BOOKS BY ROBERT ROOT-BERNSTEIN
*Discovering: Inventing and Solving Problems
at the Frontiers of Scientific Knowledge*
*Rethinking AIDS: The Tragic Cost of Premature
Consensus*

BOOK BY MICHÈLE ROOT-BERNSTEIN
*Boulevard Theater and Revolution in
Eighteenth-Century Paris*

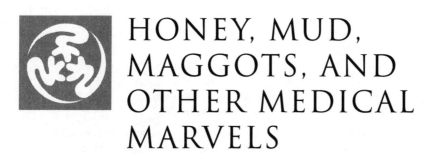

HONEY, MUD, MAGGOTS, AND OTHER MEDICAL MARVELS

*The Science Behind Folk Remedies
and Old Wives' Tales*

Robert and Michèle Root-Bernstein

Houghton Mifflin Company
Boston ❧ New York ❧ 1997

For information about permission to reproduce selections
from this book, write to Permissions, Houghton Mifflin Company,
215 Park Avenue South, New York, New York 10003.

Library of Congress Cataloging-in-Publication Data

Root-Bernstein, Robert Scott.
Honey, mud, maggots, and other medical marvels : the
science behind folk remedies and old wives' tales /
Robert and Michèle Root-Bernstein.
p.   cm.
Includes bibliographical references and index.
ISBN 0-395-82298-xx
1. Alternative medicine.   2. Traditional medicine.
I. Root-Bernstein, Michèle.   II. Title.
R733.R66   1997
615.8'8 — dc21   97-23267   CIP

Printed in the United States of America

QUM 10 9 8 7 6 5 4 3 2 1

Book design by Joyce Weston

Although this book describes a number of medically validated therapies currently used in modern hospitals that originated as folk treatments, this book should in no way be construed as recommending that laypeople practice these therapies or other folk remedies on themselves or anyone else. Medicine should be practiced only by trained medical personnel. Many folk remedies, including the therapies described in this book, involve significant risks, and some are potentially fatal. If you desire to be treated in some of the ways we describe, see a trained physician for advice and care. Please note as well that the authors are not physicians and cannot dispense medical counsel of any kind.

*Meredith and Brian, for your health,
education, and enjoyment*

ACKNOWLEDGMENTS

Allan Burdick, Courtney Clark, Harold Conn, Patrick and Maureen Dillon, Norman Kasting, Ann Kerwin, Elizabeth Knoll, Barbara Mathes, Isaac Sanday, Jerome Sullivan, Marlys and Charles Witte, and the science librarians of Michigan State University all contributed in various ways to this book. We thank them.

CONTENTS

The philosophies of one age become the absurdities of the next, and the foolishness of yesterday has become the wisdom of tomorrow.

— Sir William Osler, M.D., 1902

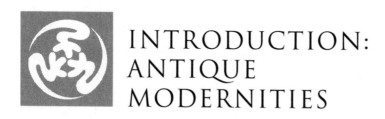

INTRODUCTION: ANTIQUE MODERNITIES

*Medicine is in a period of development of which we
the contemporaries cannot grasp the full
significance. But one thing is obvious, namely,
that what we lack is no longer facts, observations,
experiments, new treatments; it is rather the
philosophy of medicine that is going astray. It is all
too apparent that, carried away, we too much neglect
the lessons of medicine of all times and peoples.*
— B. J. Stokvis, Ph.D., 1896

IMAGINE THAT you are lying in a hospital
emergency room at a major university with a
festering wound that is beginning to turn gangrenous. The doctor
says, "First I'm going to put some maggots in there to clean out the
wound, and when they're through, I'll pack it with honey and
cover it with some cellophane. It's the latest thing. You'll be up
and about in no time."

Or perhaps the group you're traveling with has had a car
accident out in the desert. You have no medical supplies, not even
water to drink. One of your companions has a fever, and her
temperature is dangerously high; you have sustained a deep cut
that would normally require stitches. Fortunately a medical in-
tern is with you. He cleanses the wound with your urine, pulls the
edges together with safety pins, and suggests that you lick the
damaged flesh regularly to keep it moist as it heals. To treat the
woman with the raging fever, he takes out his penknife, sterilizes it

1

with a lit match, then proceeds to puncture a vein in her arm and withdraw more than a pint of blood. He claims he has just saved your lives.

Or maybe you have high blood pressure and water retention due to some liver or kidney problem. Your internist says you don't need any pills. He recommends instead that you check into a spa for a month and sit up to your neck in water for a minimum of one hour twice a day. Oh, and drink lots of the local mineral water. That should do the trick.

These scenes may sound preposterous, but they are not. They are based on treatments that have actually been used in hospital settings or emergency situations within the last few years or on treatments that have recently accrued sufficient medical backing that they could be. All of them originated as folk remedies and have been employed for generations, even millennia. That they sound utterly preposterous to us today just goes to show how completely we have lost touch with the wisdom of the past.

For thousands of years medical knowledge was reverently passed on from generation to generation. Bloodletting, bathing in mineral springs, cleansing with urine — all these practices had long therapeutic lives in both folk and learned medicines in every part of the world. Few changes were made in the care and treatment of sickness and injury from the time the ancient Egyptians, Greeks, Hindus, and Chinese wrote down their first texts through the mid-nineteenth century. Much of what was learned over this time resulted from the sharing of insights between cultures as travel and communication made the world ever smaller. Then, quite abruptly, the advent of "scientific medicine" in the later 1800s seriously undermined the unquestioned acceptance of past medical traditions. Rudyard Kipling caught the new spirit of these times when he wrote:

> Wonderful little, when all is said,
> Wonderful little our fathers knew.
> Half their remedies cured you dead —
> Most of their teaching was quite untrue . . .

Suddenly, as Henry Sigerist, a leading medical historian, put it, "the history of medicine," became "the history of errors." So great was the enthusiasm for medical breakthroughs based upon the chemical analysis of drugs, systematic record-keeping, surgical innovations, and scientific research, and so boundless the optimism in medicine's future progress, that the past seemed to hold no value either for doctors or for their patients. The consequences of this shift in medical mindset are still with us today. Indeed, it is not uncommon for medical researchers and physicians to restrict their studies to the last five or ten years of medical progress. Of the history of medicine the average person is likely to know only the tall tales of supposedly nonsensical treatments such as phlebotomy, poultices, and purges. The nonscientific roots of medicine seem ever more ridiculous and ever more obscure.

Such flippant rejection of many millennia of accumulated knowledge has its price, as does the rejection of traditional medicines from foreign cultures. Ignorance of the past has never been a firm foundation for the present. "Medical history," wrote Sigerist in 1951, "is medicine, also, today as it was in the past." The proposition is not obvious, but it can be demonstrated. In the past, both ancient and recent, in Europe and around the world, general truths are still to be found; common regimens and serendipitous cures can still be examined for present and future benefit. "Today more than ever," Sigerist said, "there is need also for medical interpretations and evaluations of the past of medicine."

This book is a serious exercise in this vein but with a lighthearted twist. What follows is an anecdotal examination of a number of medicinal remedies from long ago or across the world that have influenced and continue to influence modern medical practice. These stories run the gamut from comedy to drama to romance, from triumph to failure, from discovery to dénouement. They turn upon makeshift, foresight, curiosity, horror, hard work, and devotion. In each case, an ancient treatment we have been taught to ignore, abhor, or poke fun at is found making a comeback at the cutting edge of modern clinical practice. Separately, each tale tells of some obligation we bear toward the wisdom of other times and other places. Together they tell us that medicine's past is the key to its present and its future.

Above all, these stories spell out the evolutionary pattern of medical progress. With evolutionary theory as our guide, we can discern the biological origins of medicine and trace its subsequent cultural growth. We can look at the basic physiological urges that gave rise to primitive therapies and examine the cultural forces of selection and repression that limit the horizons of medicine. We can investigate the social pressures that encourage medical crackpots, on the one hand, and medical innovators, on the other. We can begin to understand why medical remedies of any kind must fit the practitioners' minds and spirits in order to be both efficacious and utilized. Finally, we can learn from the past evolutionary course of medicine what we must do to shape its evolution in the future. The lessons of medical history, and how we may use them, are the subject of *Honey, Mud, Maggots, and Other Medical Marvels.*

In sketching out this narrative, however, we have set severe limits on the old wives' tales and treatments we will discuss. We consider very few herbal remedies because the literature on herbal medicines and their histories is already large and compelling. One well-known academic press, CRC Publishers, has an entire ethnobotanical library. We also believe that the focus on herbal remedies has largely blinded physicians, medical historians, and the public to other branches of modern medicine that have been affected by folk wisdom. Of these, we wished to present only those treatments amply validated by recent medical practice. Our ultimate criterion has been, in fact, that accredited physicians working in established hospitals in industrialized countries use the treatment, or some historical offspring of the treatment, today. We firmly believe that medicine can benefit from folk wisdom only if the very highest clinical standards are maintained.

Our purpose is not to convince the world that folk medicine is the answer to all the limitations faced by contemporary medical science. We are all too well aware that the majority of folk treatments do not work or work less effectively than modern medicines. It would be foolish to throw out current practice without the most compelling of reasons. Rather, our purpose is to demonstrate the much more circumscribed thesis that ancient folk medicines have provided so many useful therapies that to ignore this fecund source of knowledge and practice is also foolish. We owe a profound medical debt to the past and to the multiple cultures of the world, and we should be proud to acknowledge it.

We also have an obligation to maximize medicine's adaptive response to the rapidly changing world we anticipate in the twenty-first century. Traditional medicines in non-Western countries as well as alternative medicines in Western popular culture can offer catalysts for creative change in standard clinical practice. The systematic and serious review of these practices can prime the pump of medical innovation. "Antique modernities" mark a tried and true path toward discovery and rediscovery. We owe it to our children and our children's children to make the journey, to see where we have been, where we need to go, and how we can get there.

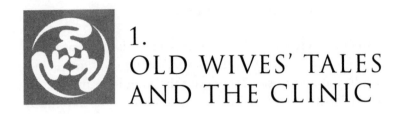

1.
OLD WIVES' TALES
AND THE CLINIC

Although constantly practiced by primitive people for thousands of years, these methods have been recently rediscovered by learned men, clothed in scientific principle, and given to the world as new.
— George Engelmann, Ph.D., 1884

ONE DAY the teenaged Edward Jenner, apprentice to the English surgeon John Ludlow, went with his master to see a man whom Ludlow diagnosed as having smallpox. Greatly feared, smallpox killed many and often left those who survived forever scarred and even blind. The usual procedure was to send the family away, quarantine the patient, and find a nurse who had already survived the disease and therefore would not catch it again. In this instance, however, one of the man's servants, a milkmaid, claimed she could take care of her sick master without harm because she had had the cowpox. Ludlow scoffed. Cowpox seriously affected cows and horses but caused only mild symptoms in human beings. They do say it protects against the smallpox, the girl replied. Stuff and nonsense, warned Ludlow. Smallpox was another disease altogether, and the milkmaid ran a serious risk of catching it. Still the girl persisted. She had already nursed people sick with smallpox and been safe, sir. Ludlow threw up his hands and allowed her to stay. Afterward Jenner asked if there might be something to this cowpox notion. Put no credence in old wives' tales, Ludlow roundly scolded his apprentice. The only safe way to prevent smallpox was variolization.

Variolization was an inoculation procedure in which pus from a very light case of smallpox, or variola, was scratched into the skin of a healthy person. Usually this person came down with a light case of smallpox, which more often than not protected against severe strains of the disease. Jenner already knew this, having been inoculated himself as a small boy. He may also have known that variolization had originated in the Orient 2000 years earlier. The practice had been observed near the beginning of the eighteenth century by Lady Mary Wortley Montagu, wife of the British ambassador to Turkey. Although she had initially been appalled by the barbarity of purposefully transmitting such a horrible disease, she had had herself and her son variolized in 1717. On her return to England she brought the practice with her and for the most part it worked, although sometimes even a light case of smallpox could scar or maim or kill a person.

Jenner was concerned. The best defense against smallpox was not without considerable risk. He was also intrigued. Variolization had been introduced to Europeans, not by a properly accredited male physician but by an untrained woman relying upon exotic ways. Perhaps a better method existed! Perhaps that better method was also to be found among the strange beliefs of untutored people! Perhaps there really was something to the local folklore that cowpox protected against smallpox, an idea that, as he began to practice on his own, he heard repeated on all sides. Jenner decided to see for himself. Despite the medical profession's disdain for old wives' tales, he began to keep track of what happened to patients who had contracted cowpox when they were later exposed to smallpox.

One of his earliest cases concerned a farmer named Joseph Merret, whom Jenner attended in 1770. Merret developed an unusually severe cowpox infection that laid him up for several days. Five years later Jenner inoculated the farmer and his family with a weakened strain of smallpox as part of a general variolization campaign. The rest of Merret's family became infected, but despite repeated inoculations, Merret did not get sick from the weakened smallpox infection. Perhaps he really was protected.

In 1785 Jenner found five more cowpox-infected farmhands and inoculated them with smallpox. None became ill. Excited by these results, Jenner summarized his six cases for the local medical society. He suggested inoculating people purposefully with cowpox to test his theory that it protected against smallpox. His fellow physicians, however, refused to entertain the notion. Folk wisdom, they told him, was dangerous nonsense.

Though discouraged, Jenner persevered, collecting more and more cases. In 1792 he treated Sarah Portlock, who had become infected with cowpox while employed as a farm servant. Portlock's daughter contracted smallpox later that year, and Sarah nursed her. Because the case was light, and Sarah had already been exposed to her daughter's case, Jenner used pus from the daughter to inoculate Sarah. Despite repeated inoculations, she did not contract smallpox. Protection again.

And so it went. Altogether Jenner accumulated more than one hundred instances of people who had had definitive cases of cowpox and had subsequently been exposed to smallpox without contracting it. Finally, during an outbreak of cowpox in 1796, Jenner took cowpox pus from the arms of Sarah Nelmes, inoculated a young boy named James Phipps with it, and a few weeks later attempted to give the Phipps boy smallpox. How Jenner got permission from Phipps's parents to perform this experiment is not recorded, but Phipps did not get smallpox. He was protected, as Jenner had predicted.

By now Jenner believed he had enough data to convince his medical colleagues that cowpox inoculations would be safer and more effective than variolization. In 1798 he asked the Royal Society of London, the premier scientific institution in Great Britain and, indeed, the world, to sponsor his results. The answer was no. Jenner had no choice but to publish his breakthrough as a pamphlet at his own expense. He subsequently endured years of unkind treatment from both colleagues and public before his ideas were finally accepted.

Today, of course, Jenner is known as the inventor of vaccination, a term derived from the latin word *vacca,* or cow. And due to his invention, smallpox itself has been eradicated worldwide. Indeed, vaccination for this and many other diseases may very well save more lives every year than any other medical procedure invented since. Jenner's discovery was surely a case in which folk wisdom yielded a nugget of truth that the modern world could hardly do without.

Another eighteenth-century physician, by the name of William Withering, also found medicine in old wives' tales. He turned an interest in the folk medicinal use of plants into the discovery of digitalis. Like Jenner, Withering was wise enough to realize what he and his profession did not know, and that was how to treat heart disease. His ignorance was brought home to him sharply by a patient he treated in 1775. The elderly woman had dropsy, a severe swelling of the lower limbs. A modern doctor would probably diagnose the cause as congestive heart failure, in which the heart pumps too feebly to maintain adequate circulation of blood. Withering knew that the woman had not long to live, and he apparently prescribed no treatment. Imagine his surprise, therefore, when a few weeks later he inquired after her health and learned that she had recovered from her illness! He asked the old woman to what she attributed her miraculous recovery. Herb tea, she replied, supplied by a neighbor renowned for curing problems that physicians often were unable to treat. Upon further questioning the old woman produced the recipe and Withering decided to test it for himself.

Withering found that the tea contained some twenty herbal ingredients. Among them he quickly identified foxglove, known botanically as *Digitalis purpurea* and a staple of folk remedies from at least the Middle Ages, as the only ingredient capable of reducing a dropsical swelling. Foxglove increased urination and vomiting, and thus, Withering reasoned, reduced the volume of blood and of fluid in the body. He began experimenting with foxglove extracts of various strengths, using them on the poor people he treated for free. And he verified that foxglove extracts were, in fact, very beneficial for almost all patients suffering from dropsy — but for different reasons than he had expected; the preparations directly stimulated the heart rate, thereby improving the circulation of the blood.

Withering collected hundreds of observations and published them in 1785 in *An Account of the Foxglove and Some of Its Medical Uses.* As a result of publicity caused by Charles Darwin's grandfather's claiming the discovery for his prematurely deceased son, the use of foxglove, or digitalis, for congestive heart failure was quickly established. Today it is still widely prescribed for the same purpose. Indeed, although the chemical makeup of digitalis is now known, the common foxglove plant and closely related species continue to be the basic source from which pharmaceutical companies extract the drug and its derivatives. Nature sometimes turns out to be a better chemist than human chemists, just as old wives sometimes turn out to be better pharmacists than the professionals.

If Jenner and Withering were unique, we would not have much of a narrative, but they are not. Despite the tremendous advances made by synthetic chemists and pharmacologists in the modern era of antibiotics, chemotherapies, and anesthetics, much of our pharmacopoeia — our collection of drugs and medicinal preparations — and a good deal of our medical technique and expertise, too, have been acquired from folk practice. The medical historian Erwin Ackerknecht has, in fact, characterized the eighteenth century as a period in which the breakdown of social barriers and the rise of the middle classes in Europe lowered intellectual barriers separating learned medicine from that of everyday folk. Knowledge seeped slowly but steadily from untrained practitioners to medical professionals such as Jenner and Withering and back again.

Cowpox protection and digitalis were only two of dozens of discoveries arising from this process. The medicinal use of cod liver oil began as a Scandinavian folk remedy for rickets, scrofulas, and other wasting diseases, including tuberculosis. The oil's active ingredients were eventually identified as vitamins A and D, which are now known to be effective against the very diseases for which cod liver oil was most commonly prescribed in the past. Another worthy folk practice was the ingestion of fresh fruit, especially citrus, to prevent scurvy, the efficacy of which was demonstrated in controlled studies by the Scottish physician James Lind in 1747. The active ingredient, vitamin C, was discovered two hundred years later.

Folk wisdom outside of Europe was also mined for medical gold. Andean Indians had employed cinchona bark for centuries before Spanish explorers first encountered the "fever tree," from which the antimalarial drug quinine was eventually extracted. During the nineteenth century many other "discoveries" based upon "primitive" medical traditions made their appearance in the Western medical canon. Among these the use of willow bark, a source of the salicylic acid upon which aspirin is based, has been traced back 3500 years to an ancient Egyptian document known as the Ebers Papyrus. The use of dried sap from the opium poppy has a similarly long medical history, long predating the isolation from opium of morphine, a stronger painkiller, by Frederick Sertürner in 1806. And ouabain, a steroid hormone employed against cardiac arrhythmias, had been used from time out of mind by East African tribes for both medical purposes and, in much more concentrated doses, as a poison for their spears and arrows.

The process of discovery continues to this day. Taxol, a recently discovered anticancer agent derived from the Pacific yew tree, has been a part of concoctions used by Native Americans for countless generations. An ancient Chinese chemical remedy for fever has yielded the active ingredient arsenic trioxide, which has been used for decades in veterinary medicine to treat parasitic and blood diseases. Recent research reveals that arsenic trioxide is the most effective treatment yet found for a rare blood cancer called acute promyelocytic leukemia.

Modern medical science has substantiated many other common folk beliefs as well. Perhaps you have heard that drinking cranberry juice may help treat a urinary tract infection. Indeed it may, and so might blueberries. Pharmacologists have recently isolated a compound from both berries that interferes with the ability of bacteria to attach to the bladder. And if your great-aunt ever suggested placing a brewed tea bag on your eye to treat a sty, she was probably right; black teas have been found to contain active antibiotics. The Chinese and Japanese have long recommended green tea for many ills, and recent research has shown that it may indeed have some anticancer activity. Almost certainly it protects teeth from decay. The Chinese have an old saying: "When you eat a sweet, drink green tea." Someday a group of chemicals called hexanes, the cavity fighters found in green tea, may end up in your toothpaste.

The list of efficacious folk medicines is so long that it would take an entire book just to summarize them. In fact, in 1970 Virgil Vogel studied the origins of drugs then listed in two standard guides, the *Pharmacopoeia of the United States of America* and the *National Formulary*. He found some 120 substances that had been used previously by Indians of North and Central America. Dr. Maurice Gordon found further that at least 59 of these had not been known to Europeans until they came into contact with American Indians. If we assume, as further evidence suggests, an equal number of drugs originating in other cultures around the world, the list of medically validated folk cures that have become part of the modern pharmacopoeia is immensely long. It has been estimated that as many as half of the drugs (prescription and over-the-counter) currently available to physicians in the West began as old wives' tales or concoctions used by so-called primitive peoples. According to a tally kept by one pharmaceutical company, of the 121 prescription drugs currently derived just from plant materials (as opposed to chemical synthesis), "74 percent came from following up native folklore claims."

Medicine has benefited not only from the drug lore of primitive and ancient peoples but also from their knowledge of surgical techniques and disease processes. Ancient Egyptian medical papyri show that broken bones were immobilized with bandages soaked in cream and bean flour or other materials that hardened as they dried. Such casts were used for thousands of years before the invention of plaster of Paris. The Edwin Smith Surgical Papyrus, which dates to 1700 B.C., describes the even more difficult and delicate treatment of a broken nose by packing it with soft material and covering with an adhesive plaster — just as we might do today. And recent analysis of surgical reconstructive methods in India 1500 years before Christ has found that Hindu surgeons had worked out all of the basic procedures now used for nasal reconstruction.

European contact with the Americas revealed that native Indians were hundreds, if not thousands, of years ahead of their more civilized counterparts in the medical treatment of childbirth. Not only did the Amerindians use various methods to alleviate pain (including alcohol and narcotic drugs and, in severe cases, partial suffocation to relax the mother), but they worked out the basic methods for expelling a withheld placenta long before European doctors did. George Engelmann, a nineteenth-century physician who made a special study of American Indian medical practices, remarked that all too often his contemporaries thought they had invented treatments that he found to be "as old as the world."

Native Americans had also realized by the time Europeans invaded their lands that whatever caused putrefaction in a warrior's wounds or caused illness in a woman who had given birth was transmissible to others. They therefore isolated the injured and newborns and their mothers in individual huts. Each patient was cared for by a single individual who was forbidden to treat anyone else at the same time. As a result, puerperal, or childbirth, fever was very rare among Indians, even while it decimated women of European descent. And while hundreds of thousands, perhaps even millions, of men died during our frontier wars and the Civil War of infected wounds, or had to have limbs amputated due to gangrene, physicians in the Old West noted that very few Indians similarly injured in battle suffered the same fate.

Many European physicians believed that the Indians' treatment of wounds was far superior to their own. This opinion was common enough that it fueled the popular rage for "Indian Medicine Wagons" and "Indian Medicine Shows" in the last decades of the nineteenth century. Unfortunately, only the medicines were mimicked and not the equally important procedures of isolation and individualized care. Otherwise Western medicine might have recognized earlier that centralizing medical care also centralizes the sources of infection and makes their spread more efficient. As the Indians proved, one does not need to know about germs in order to make crucial observations and act rationally upon them to save lives.

A good case can, in fact, be made that medical science might have understood various modes of disease transmission substantially sooner than it did if researchers had paid attention to folk wisdom. Drawing on local tales, the Cuban physician Carlos Finlay suggested that yellow fever was carried by mosquitoes several decades before Walter Reed finally thought to test the insight in 1901. Similarly, the explorer Richard F. Burton wrote in the 1850s that the Somali people blamed mosquitoes for other fever-causing diseases, "from the fact that mosquitoes and fevers become formidable about the same time." Forty years elapsed, however, before Sir Ronald Ross traced the spread of malaria to the pesky insects, thereby earning a Nobel Prize.

In these cases intuition was initially rejected as "superstition." But sometimes superstition deserves careful study. If but one physician had seized upon Finlay's suggestion or Burton's footnote, as Withering seized upon the tea that cured an old woman or as Jenner followed up on the chance remark of a milkmaid, how much sooner might yellow fever and malaria have yielded to public health controls? More important, how many equally revealing clues from odd sources are being overlooked at this very moment because they do not fit our preconceived notions of disease causation or treatment? Think about Augusto and Michaela Odone, whose son lay dying from amyotrophic leukodystrophy, or ALD.

With no medical training, these well-educated parents developed an unusual dietary treatment, "Lorenzo's oil," that arrested the progress of that debilitating disease — despite hostility from the medical community. Some physicians have adopted Lorenzo's oil as a way to slow the progress of ALD while they continue to look for a cure. But as a society we are no more likely to acknowledge the insights of dedicated laymen than we are to accept those of untutored folk.

This is not to say that such insights are always overlooked or scorned by experts. Indeed, a generation ago, a purposeful search for medical folk wisdom was undertaken by Dr. Richard Schultes, a director of the Botanical Museum of Harvard University, and his doctoral student Siri von Reis Altschul, subsequently a professor of pharmacology. Schultes spent more than a decade after World War II exploring the wilderness of the Amazon River Basin and gathering plant specimens and tribal lore concerning their uses. Altschul, meanwhile, delved into the centuries-old collections and records of the Arnold Arboretum and Gray Herbarium of Harvard, where she found hundreds upon hundreds of anecdotes concerning the medicinal or food uses of little-known plants. Together these investigators found that related species of plants from very different locations were often used by the local cultures for the same medical purposes.

Modern chemical research has identified in many of these plants active compounds that have served as the bases of new experimental drugs. When Michael Balick, director of the Institute of Economic Botany of the New York Botanical Garden, sampled the Garden's plant specimens from around the world for extracts that could be used against human immunodeficiency virus (HIV), he found that plants identified by native healers as being "powerful" were four times more likely to have general antiviral activity than those chosen at random. Several compounds derived from these plants are now being developed for further testing by the National Cancer Institute. That is pretty impressive, since none of the native healers (many interviewed by plant collectors more than a century ago) had ever heard of viruses or of AIDS.

Given these surprising results, growing numbers of researchers have in recent years focused on culling folk medicines for modern medical insights. The ethnobotanist Paul Alan Cox, for instance, has spent the last decade gathering the medical knowledge of local healers in Tonga, Fiji, Australia, Africa, Costa Rica, and, most often and by preference, Samoa. Some of his botanical specimens have already yielded disease-fighting drugs. Nor is Cox alone. There are enough professionals interested in non-Western medical traditions to support journals of ethnobotany, ethnomedicine, and ethnopharmacology, as well as journals and books on alternative medicines. Schultes, now the old man of the field, has recently founded an ethnobotanical conservation institute to centralize such efforts.

One pharmaceutical company, based in San Marcos, California, actually specializes in tracking down folk cures and turning them into modern medicines. Shaman Pharmaceuticals has already delivered several drugs derived from ethnobotanical sources to clinical trial. These recent successes have spurred some two hundred pharmaceutical companies and research institutions worldwide into investigating plants as sources of useful drugs. Traditional medicines serve as a starting point. Even the United States government has gotten into the act with the recent founding of the Office of Alternative and Non-Traditional Medicine within the Department of Health and Human Services. Since a majority of Americans self-treat with remedies originating outside the modern medical tradition prior to visiting a physician, it is high time that we study folk medicines and alternative therapies more thoroughly. If nothing else, physicians need to understand the treatments their patients choose to use and why they do so.

Whether alternative medical treatments are valid is, of course, a different question altogether. Some are undoubtedly nonsensical, if not downright harmful, as we discuss in Chapter 17, "Crackpots and Panaceas." Others no doubt contain a grain of truth as useful as those recognized by Jenner and Withering. As long as we remain ignorant of the facts of each case, we cannot distinguish between the two.

It will not be easy to overcome our ignorance. No one, least of all a trained professional, is comfortable with the unfamiliar, as many of our examples here and in the following chapters will show. Most physicians reacted negatively to Jenner's idea of vaccination and to Withering's foxglove tea. They ignored what the American Indians knew about close quarters and contagion, what Finlay and others suggested about insects and fever, what the Odones learned about diet and ALD. And, as we will see in subsequent chapters, physicians have turned up their noses at the medical use of maggots, sugar, and leeches, pooh-poohed deepwater bathing, and gagged at the thought (and smell) of pus. Resistance to innovation is natural, deeply ingrained in all of us. Consider your own reactions to the following case.

Imagine yourself a physician. A farmer comes into your office and tells you he thinks he has heartburn. You ask whether he has ever been evaluated for a heart condition, which can have similar symptoms and would be much more serious. He says yes, but the problem has been taken care of. When you inquire further, he reveals that ten years earlier he was diagnosed as having "heart palpitations" and was put on a drug that sounds like "quinine." You interpret that to mean he had a heart arrhythmia treated by quinidine. After taking the drug for a few months, the symptoms went away, so the farmer stopped taking the drug. Then the symptoms came back. The farmer no longer had the drug, so he just bore the pain and went off to do his daily chores. In the course of his work, he had to replace a downed electrical wire that ran around his pasture to keep the cows from straying. As he stood in the wet grass, he grasped the wire in both hands without thinking. Instantly he felt a shock and found himself lying on his back. His heart problem had disappeared, though. So every time the farmer felt his symptoms returning, he'd shock himself on purpose. It was so effective, he even ran a line from the fence into his basement for easier access to his unusual remedy.

Do you take this man's story seriously? Is he a jerk or a

genius? Would you try his treatment on yourself or your other patients? Should you search for a possible ulcer, or should you suggest psychiatric treatment instead? Might he have made up this story to pull your leg, or is it for real?

The farmer is for real, and the story is told by Dr. Jerry H. Berke of Acton, Massachusetts, who thinks the farmer was extraordinarily clever: "I most probably would have dismissed his tale as so much colorful folklore . . . ," he writes, "if I hadn't known that an electric shock passed across the chest could effectively resolve cardiac arrhythmias." The farmer had simply reinvented for himself a treatment that has been known to physicians for decades and that is the basis for the heroic efforts you see on TV when the emergency-room physician claps the paddles onto the chest of a fibrillating heart patient and yells, "Clear!"

Dr. Berke's punchline however, is this: "I have to wonder what other potentially useful therapeutic modalities have been similarly dismissed by me and my learned colleagues." And well he might. Norman Kasting, whose foray into the history of medicine we will discuss in Chapter 6, recounts his own initial refusal to consider medical evidence simply because it originated in the past:

> I was often given the advice to familiarize myself with the works of the early pioneers in my field. My supervisors were determined that I should gain some perspective on my own research. At first I paid relatively little heed to their kindly admonitions, scarcely believing that research done 20 years ago, much less 100 years ago, could be very meaningful to current research problems. The mere mention of papers from 1883 conjured up images of aging and slightly senile medical historians cloistered in darkened rooms full of dusty old manuscripts and muttering medieval words such as "phlogiston" or "plethora" to themselves. I wondered how relevant this old stuff could be when they didn't even have oxygen analyzers, data acquisition systems, oscilloscopes, or radioimmunoassays.

At first Kasting's forays into the archives seemed to confirm his preconceptions, leaving him with the feeling "that I was wasting valuable time that could otherwise be used to push back the frontiers of knowledge." Such feelings are prevalent. Surely the laboratory is where discoveries are made, not the library or the ethnographic records of some primitive shaman or the recipes of half-educated housewives or the cockamamie story of some farmer! But much of the dis-ease with the past and the unfamiliar comes from not knowing what to look for or how to go about it. Once one becomes "fluent" in library skills, interviewing, and in the disconcerting and sometimes baroque disquisitions of laymen, new worlds of experience suddenly become accessible. "It wasn't long," Kasting writes, "before I discovered just how useful these carefully written chronicles of early physiology could be."

The dialogue between modern medicine and folk practice "works" because they both have, in fact, a common goal. Every culture on earth has needed medicines and medical treatments, and all have experimented with the resources available to them. As a result, a process of trial and error has been going on for thousands — perhaps hundreds of thousands — of years. Therapies that worked were retained and passed down from generation to generation. Those that did not work were discarded, and something else was tried instead. Ancient remedies that have withstood this test of time, especially those that have survived in many cultures around the world have, we believe, a high probability of effectiveness. Once we understand how they work, these remedies can be used to enhance the range and flexibility of modern medicine.

Like Kasting, the best professionals recognize that regardless of formal credentials, anyone in any culture who is committed to solving an outstanding medical problem may have an intuition that leads to a promising treatment or cure. Indeed, given the extraordinarily limited means available to contemporary native healers and past practitioners in terms of knowledge, technology, and technique, the results they have achieved are often quite astounding. Few of us are as inventive or insightful as the medical innovators hidden in the past, the bush, the farm, or even the urban jungle! But we can push the frontiers of our own medicine by culling what is useful from the accumulated wisdom of shamans and laymen alike. The road from old wives' tales to the modern clinic is still being paved with solutions to many of mankind's most pressing medical problems.

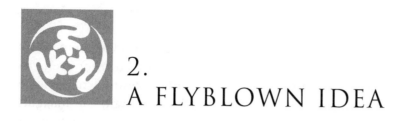

2.
A FLYBLOWN IDEA

*While it is natural to look to future research to
provide new modalities of therapy, one should not
overlook successes of the past. One such technique of
the pre-antibiotic era for treatment of suppurative
infections was the use of maggots.*
— Karl Lawrence Horn, M.D.; Albert H. Cobb,
Jr., M.D.; and George A. Gates, M.D., 1976

MEDICAL TREATMENTS are rarely
pretty, at least to the untrained or unac-
customed eye. When they come in unusual forms and from unusual sources, even physicians can be shocked. Dr. William A.
Nolen learned this lesson early in the 1950s at Bellevue Hospital
in New York City.

On his first day as a resident in the outpatient department,
Nolen was taken in hand by a nurse known as Riley, a no-nonsense
type who set him straight on the alcoholics and drug addicts who
came to the clinic with leg ulcers. "Be tough," she told him. The
first couple of patients needed only a dressing change, a third
required admission to the hospital. Then Riley began unwrapping
the bandaged leg of a man covered in filth and grime. "As she
took away the last layer of gauze," Nolen recalled, "I saw, crawling
around on three inches of bare bone, a swarm of maggots. I almost
vomited." Riley, though, had seen it all. She calmly dosed the
maggots with ether, causing them to roll up and out of the wound.
What she said next shocked Nolen almost as much as his first sight

of the crawling mass itself: "Those maggots sure keep an ulcer clean."

Nolen, who had been too distressed to do more than glance at the wound, looked more closely. Sure enough, the maggots seemed to have eaten only dead tissue, leaving the ulcer looking "red and healthy." Even so, Nolen needed a breath of fresh air. Since ancient times the infestation of human flesh by maggots has been considered a repugnant affliction. Riley, however, had pointed out a phenomenon repeatedly observed, forgotten, and rediscovered over the centuries: sometimes maggots do good in a wound rather than harm. "Not much to look at," Riley conceded, "but they do the job."

Those maggots, of course, were the larvae of flies that lay their eggs on raw or rotting flesh. And it is likely that their beneficial medical effects on open wounds were first observed in prehistoric times. We know that in the early part of this century the Ngemba tribe of New South Wales, Australia, commonly used maggots to cleanse suppurating or gangrenous wounds; the aborigines traced the treatment back to their remote ancestors. The same may be true of certain isolated hill people in Burma, observed around World War II placing maggots on wounds and then covering them with mud and wet grass. Ancient records suggest that the Maya Indians of Central America ceremonially exposed dressings of beef blood to the sun before applying them to certain superficial tumors. After a few days the dressings were expected to pulsate with maggots. The evidence, though slim, is tantalizing. For thousands of years, perhaps, in areas of the world as far apart as the Americas, Asia, and Australia, people have used maggots as medicine.

We need not tramp so far afield as the bush or the rain forest, however, to find comprehension of a beneficial association between man and maggot. At the battle of Saint-Quentin, France, in 1557, the barber-surgeon Ambroise Paré observed firsthand that "the wounds of the hurt people were greatly stincking, and full of *wormes* with gangrene and putrifaction." Paré did not know that the "wormes" were fly larvae; he believed that they spontaneously generated from the "corruption" of rotting flesh. But he did treat at least one traumatic maggot-infested wound in which "the patient recovered beyond all men's expectation." This is considered the first European recognition of the maggot's medical industry.

It was by no means the last. Over the next three hundred years the efficacy of maggots was sporadically noticed, most especially by Napoléon's famous military surgeon, Dominique-Jean Larrey. During the French expedition in Egypt, the majority of injured soldiers with suppurating wounds were, according to Larrey, "much annoyed by the worms or larvae of the blue fly, peculiar to that climate." Larrey and his medical staff tried unsuccessfully to convince the soldiers that the maggots merely "cut short the process of nature" and promoted healing by eating the dead and dying flesh. Nevertheless, when they changed dressings the medical men made every effort to cleanse the wounds and prevent reinfestation.

Obviously, it is one thing to notice that maggots serendipitously aid in the healing process of severe wounds. It is another to use them deliberately as therapeutic agents. Although Australian aborigines, Burmese hill people, and the Maya Indians seem to have made the leap long ago, in Western medicine the purposeful use of maggots to clean wounds dates back only to the mid-nineteenth century in France and in the United States. The American experience was again tied to fields of battle, for during the Civil War myiasis, or natural infestation of wounds, was a common, if awful, sight. Many army surgeons recognized the maggots' beneficial effects, but a Confederate physician, John Forney Zacharias, was the first to use maggots purposefully to remove the gangrenous flesh of his hospital patients. "During my service . . . at Danville, Virginia," he wrote, "I first used maggots to remove the decayed tissue in hospital gangrene and with eminent satisfaction. In a single day they would clean a wound much better than any agents we had at our command. I used them afterwards at various places. I am sure I saved many lives by their use, escaped septicaemia, and had rapid recoveries."

Subsequent therapeutic use of maggots was hindered, however, by several factors. To begin with, there are some 80,000 known species of flies, at least four large families of which feed on animal protein during their larval stage. For every species of maggot that feeds only on dead and dying tissue, there is another that feeds indiscriminantly on both dead or living flesh and yet another that feeds primarily on living flesh. Unfortunately, a number of these flies and their maggots look very much the same. Without some means to distinguish among them, the deliberate use of maggots could do harm as easily as good.

Moreover, even the right flies and their maggots can infect a wound. The discovery of germs and the invention of the germ theory of disease by Louis Pasteur and Robert Koch during the 1880s altered forever the physician's willingness to introduce contaminating agents into the body. The germ theory was quickly followed by the development of antiseptic technique, revolutionizing the treatment of wounds. Under the best conditions, the use of chemical dressings and bandaging procedures significantly improved recovery. By the late nineteenth century no one in the medical profession actively promoted the purposeful use of maggots, though some evidence exists that accidental infestation of wounds in hospital wards was both tolerated and appreciated.

Then World War I introduced a new generation of physicians to types of wounds and conditions of filth few had ever experienced. Unless the wounded received immediate surgical care, virulent infection set in. Antiseptic techniques were not enough; mortality among the wounded reached 75 percent. Given these desperate circumstances more than a few military surgeons noticed that in cases of delayed treatment, those wounds did best that had been naturally infested with fly larvae. At least one suggested "raising a brood of tame maggots," a piece of advice considered a jest, although rumor had it that many American physicians at the front really were attempting to induce maggot infestation. One surgeon, William Baer, took his wartime observations to heart. Two men under his care had lain on the battlefield for seven days. By the time they reached the hospital their very severe wounds were crawling with maggots. Yet the men had no fever, no infection, and no gangrene. When the maggots were removed, Baer saw "the most beautiful pink granulation tissue that you can imagine." The wounds were actually healing.

Baer never forgot that sight, even after he returned to the hygienic conditions of peacetime medicine. As clinical professor of orthopedic surgery at the Johns Hopkins University School of Medicine, he specialized in osteomyelitis, a debilitating and painful infection of the bones. In many cases the pus-filled, ulcerating sores became chronic, lasting from four to ten years and more; the duration of the disease was all the more disturbing because so many of the sick were children. Moreover, the standard therapy of surgical debridement — the cutting away of infected or dying tissue — followed by rounds of antiseptic dressing was all too often ineffective. Multiple surgical interventions were necessary and as with war wounds, the eventual mortality was high. In 1929, after mulling the problem over for a decade, Baer decided to use maggots in his civilian practice.

Baer began by recreating the natural conditions of infestation he had witnessed on the battlefield. He selected twenty-one patients with chronic osteomyelitis, opened their lesions surgically, removing as much dead tissue as possible, and packed the wounds to stop the bleeding. No chemical aseptic agents were used. The following day he filled the wounds with what he called a "viable antiseptic" — as many maggots of the local blowfly as the wounds would hold. The maggots were replaced every four days for six or seven weeks, during which time dead and dying tissue was eaten away and healthy new granulation tissue began to grow. The maggots not only did a better job of debridement than the surgeons, they actually seemed to foster the healing process. There was no purulent odor, no pus, no scar tissue. The bacterial count diminished rapidly, and the wound turned a healthy alkaline. At the end of two months all twenty-one cases were completely healed. Baer's maggot trial had proved to be the quickest and most successful treatment of chronic osteomyelitis then known to medical science.

Baer died two years later in 1931, but not before convincing many skeptical physicians that maggots could provide a scientifically sound and medically palatable therapy. The two concerns went hand in hand. To allay the disgust of patients and staff, Baer constructed bulky mesh cages for the wounds, thus confining the maggots and hiding them from view. The continuous movement of the maggots caused an intense itching, which Baer relieved by dressing the skin around the wound. When several of the patients being treated came down with clinical tetanus, Baer immediately recognized the problem of contamination from naturally raised maggots. He and his associates began breeding blowflies in the laboratory and worked out meticulous procedures for sterilizing their eggs for clinical use. Enthusiastic medical colleagues soon adapted and improved on the Baer technique in their own clinics. Government entomologists helped by identifying fly species and learning their physiology and optimal culture; everyone wanted to avoid the horrible mistake made in one hospital that accidentally bred screwworm flies, whose larvae ate living, not necrotic or dying, flesh.

Not surprisingly, many surgeons adamantly refused to give maggots a chance, despite suggestions that the treatment by some other name — larval therapy, for instance — would smell sweeter. Part of their resistance was due to the fact that no one really knew for sure how maggots managed to heal wounds. Various hypotheses postulated that they mechanically irritated wound tissue, that they stimulated the production of blood serum, that they secreted some metabolic "active principle" — all with beneficial effect. In the hopes that the active principle could be extracted and used independently of the maggots themselves, larvae were ground into solution to produce wound dressings and "vaccines" inoculated under the skin. Further research isolated allantoin, urea, and ammonium bicarbonate in maggot excretions, and dressings made of these substances did have beneficial effects on wounds. No evidence whatsoever vindicated the maggot "vaccine," and the idea quickly got lost in the hundred or more papers written on maggot therapy between 1930 and 1940.

In the end, efforts to sanitize the maggot, both literally and figuratively, met with success. Within a few years of Baer's first trial, live maggots were being used in more than three hundred hospitals in Canada and the United States. Surgeons abroad began to take notice. A dentist in New Jersey, desperate to join the bandwagon, announced his impractical intention to use maggots in root-canal procedures. And at least two pharmaceutical houses, including Lederle Laboratories, began to mass-produce germ-free maggots for clinical use. Lederle even advertised their new "product" in the *Journal of the American Medical Association*. Despite its repugnant associations, the maggot worked better — 38 percent better, one physician reported — than any other known therapy to heal chronic festering wounds of flesh and bone.

It seemed that the maggot had taken its rightful place within the medical pharmacopoeia, but new medical developments intervened. The various sulfa drugs developed in the mid-1930s began making inroads in the treatment of wounds. By 1944 Howard Florey and Ernst Chain had figured out how to mass-produce Alexander Fleming's penicillin, a truly viable antiseptic. The three won the Nobel Prize for their work, which ushered in the era of antibiotics. With it came a virtual extinction of purposeful maggot therapy. Scientific research on the medicinal value of maggots, so vigorous in the early 1930s, fell silent by the end of the decade. For some forty years the only reminder of maggot therapy was a small amount of research on the activity of larval secretions and the infrequent notice by physicians such as William Nolen of the results of natural wound infestation. It may come as a surprise, therefore, that maggots are being used once more.

The reasons are simple. As powerful as antibiotics are, they have their limitations. Increasing numbers of patients are developing infections that do not respond to any available antibiotic or antiseptic regimen. Sometimes the problem is antibiotic-resistant strains of microbes. Sometimes it is a severe pressure sore or other uncontrollable ulceration. And sometimes it is a failed immune system, so weakened by chronic disease or severe trauma that it cannot work with antibiotics to wipe out infection. In all these situations, without the help of effective bacterial control, every effort to cut away necrotic tissue is met with its continual re-appearance. Life-threatening, festering wounds resistant to modern therapeutic practice are the result.

Such infections are costly in terms of both dollars and lives. The treatment of ulceration from a single pressure sore can cost between $30,000 and $70,000 and may require a stay of one to six months in the hospital. Moreover, multiple blood transfusions are typically needed with repeated debridements. Pressure sores result in approximately 60,000 deaths annually in the United States, and that figure takes into account only one of the major causes of chronic ulceration.

For these reasons maggot therapy has been resurrected yet again. Some rediscovery of its use, like William Nolen's, has occurred by accident. In 1984 an eighty-eight-year-old woman wandered into the emergency room of the San Francisco General Hospital Medical Center with a cheek wound filled with maggots. She had developed a facial tumor that had become necrotic, but her vision was so poor that she had not noticed. The maggot infestation had occurred quite by chance, but the woman's doctors, with her consent, allowed the larvae to finish the job they had begun. A week later the wound was closed surgically, and the woman recovered without further incident. These doctors noted that what had happened by accident could very well be turned to account.

Accident also piqued the curiosity of Drs. Edward Pechter and Ronald Sherman, two physicians who have instituted the deliberate use of maggots. Both men were at the University of California, Los Angeles, Medical Center during the 1980s when a patient came in with a leg wound crawling with worms. After their initial disgust they, like William Baer before them, noticed that healthy, infection-free tissue was growing into the wound. Excited by the clinical implications, they wrote several articles, which renewed general interest in the subject. For Pechter it was a passing fancy, but Sherman became a proselyte.

Sherman's fascination with maggots came naturally. As an undergraduate, he had earned a degree in entomology and had, in his words, "always been interested in the therapeutic uses for insects." Now at the Veterans Administration Hospital Medical Center in Long Beach, California, he has established an insectary to grow maggots for clinical use. He and his colleagues have done the first controlled study demonstrating that maggot therapy significantly increases the rate of healing of chronic pressure sores with much less cost and bother than the usual regimen of repeated surgeries and antibiotic treatments. Moreover, maggots often accomplish what typical regimens cannot. Sherman has also successfully treated cases like Harold Taylor's gangrenous leg, which if treated in the usual way would probably have required amputation. As Mr. Taylor says, "I tell you my thoughts were, I don't want to lose my leg, let's take every shot . . . Once in a while you could feel gnawing or scratching, but it didn't bother me." He thinks maggots are great.

So do an increasing number of others. More and more doctors are using what is euphemistically being called MT (for maggot therapy) or, even more cleverly, "biosurgery." Some, like Dr. John Church of Oxford, England, are following Sherman's lead and setting up their own insectaries so that they, too, can treat such difficult cases on a regular basis. Over the last twenty years maggots have been introduced into the festering wounds of people suffering from severe mastoiditis, necrotic tumors, gangrenous wounds and skin infections, burns, severe lacerations, and non-healing ulcers.

No doubt about it, maggots have earned their place in modern medicine by curing hopeless cases when all other treatments have failed. But let's be honest. No matter how effective maggots are, most of us probably look upon their use with about as much enthusiasm as Dr. Nolen did at first sight. In fact, the modern literature on maggot therapy is rather forthright about the response of patients and hospital personnel alike. Jane Petro, a surgeon at New York Medical College who uses maggots for treating necrotic tumors and burns, has noted that squeamishness is the main reason that maggot therapy is "only used on people who are in very bad shape. . . . It just goes back to the disgust factor."

Laurence Beck, chief of internal medicine at Georgetown University Medical Center in Washington D.C., has called biosurgery "gross." Certainly, compared with swallowing a pill or getting stuck with a needle, putting "wormes" in wounds seems as antiquated and repulsive as letting blood or drawing pus. Yet, as Nurse Riley said, they do the job. And when it comes down to losing your leg or letting some little larvae have a munch, that job counts.

Maggot therapy is only one of many anachronous treatments that are unexpectedly making comebacks in modern forms. To turn an old saying inside out, "All that's gold does not glitter." Many despised practices from the past harbor nuggets of wisdom at the core. If we can overcome our knee-jerk responses, we can benefit from the accumulated experience of long-forgotten or ignored medicine. After all, maggot therapy didn't turn out to be such a flyblown idea, did it?

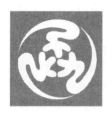

3.
SWEET TREAT(MENT)

The therapeutic potential of uncontaminated, pure honey is grossly underutilized. It is widely available in most communities and although the mechanism of action of several of its properties remains obscure and needs further investigation, the time has now come for conventional medicine to lift the blinds off this "traditional remedy" and give it its due recognition.

— A. Zumla, M.D., and A. Lulat, M.D., 1989

PARALYZED for several years, a young man in the small Mexican village of Ajoya suffers from horrendous bedsores, just the type of problem for which Ronald Sherman might prescribe maggots. But the local healer, Martín, treats the patient quite differently. Because, he says, it is cleaner in the fresh air than inside the hut, he places the young man on a table outdoors. Then Martín pulls down the patient's pants and examines the half-dozen sores, some of them so badly infected that they have delved holes all the way to the bone. These holes are big enough to stick a finger into, but it is clear from the tissue surrounding them that they were once much larger, the size of a child's fist. Martín must be doing something right; the sores are healing.

Martín cares for the people of Ajoya under the auspices of David Werner, a specialist in health care in rural communities and developing countries and recipient of a fellowship from the

MacArthur Foundation. Ajoya, like many other poor villages in Mexico, does not have any doctors, and none are within easy reach. To help rectify the situation, Werner established Project Projimo, which fosters the use of indigenous healing methods by training and supporting people like Martín in folk medicine. The results are being filmed for a documentary series on traditional medical practices by Philip Singer, a professor of Health Behavioral Sciences and Anthropology at Oakland University in Rochester, Michigan. Singer studies folk medicine and has come to observe Martín's methods.

No high-tech equipment or fancy medicines are to be found in the poverty-stricken desert around Ajoya. Martín uses simple things. First, he says, you clean the sores with iodine, or Betadine if it is available, and boiled water. He demonstrates, washing large amounts of pus out of one or two of the worst sores. Then, he continues, you "put on a mixture of sugar and honey instead of using antibiotic ointment. . . . The concentration of so much sweet — the honey and the sugar — the osmotic power that it has, no bacteria can survive. That's an antibiotic, you can think of it. By putting sugar on, it sucks from the muscle the bad liquid that is in the tissue, so that it dehydrates the tissue around the wound. Another good thing about it is that it makes the muscle grow, so that it will grow and you don't have to have surgery or special techniques to do it." Martín illustrates by pointing to the shiny new skin of sores that have already healed as a result of earlier treatments.

While Martín continues to talk, he mixes up his concoction of honey and sugar and slathers it into the infected wounds with a sterile instrument. At this point you realize how really deep some of the infections are, as the instrument disappears into the paralyzed man's gluteus maximus. You also realize the miracle that the healed sores represent. Imagine having several holes in your buttocks the size of small fists and having them not only heal, but heal in such a way that there is no indentation or muscle loss, and no surgery is required!

Singer asks, "Where did you get this idea of honey and sugar?"

Martín hesitates. "I don't know where it came from."

"Is it an old folk remedy?"

"I believe so."

"When you show this to Western doctors, what do they say?"

Martín chooses his words carefully. "Uh . . . They have to, if they are going to have the nerve to criticize, come up with a better idea to do it better. Since they don't come up with a better idea, they don't usually say much."

The folk healer's answer assumes two unstated points about what constitutes a "better idea." One is that these Western doctors would have to come up with an *economically* viable alternative. Honey and sugar are cheap and available; high-tech medicines are not. So if people want to criticize, they should come up with a treatment that is equally cheap. That would be no mean feat.

But just as importantly, a better alternative would have to be more efficacious. Any doctor who has had to treat chronic suppurating sores such as those suffered by the paralyzed young man knows that even the best Western medicines cannot compete with Martín's sugar-honey mixture in terms of what doctors call "patient outcome." Even those with access to the very best medical facilities and procedures could not treat this patient any better than Martín, and few could claim to do as well. Bedsores and other infections due to impaired circulation associated with paralysis, prolonged bed rest, complications of diabetes, burn recovery, and various other conditions present the most difficult medical problems, even in the best of conditions, even with maggots. Healing of the sort that Martín has demonstrated is very rare, especially without surgery.

Naturally this raises questions. Is Martín for real or is he perchance a quack or, even worse, a fraud? Has an unsuspecting Singer been taken in? Is Werner misusing his MacArthur Fellowship to support Martín and similarly uneducated and perhaps dangerous folk healers? Or is there, in fact, some validity to this bold remedy? Might it actually work?

The same questions that come to mind with regard to Martín's honey-sugar mixture must be raised with respect to any cure claimed by someone who has not formally satisfied the criteria of modern clinical practice. Whether we are dealing with advice from our grandmother, the herbal healer down the road, the student visiting from some exotic foreign country, an anthropologist who has recorded the practices of some remote tribe, or a historical figure writing of medicine as it was practiced a hundred or a thousand years ago, we must be wary. But we must not be so wary that we lose all sense of humility. People survived for hundreds of thousands of years without modern antibiotics, and it is worth thinking about how that was possible.

Contrary to what we might expect, mankind has made use of effective antiseptics and healing promoters at least since the beginnings of recorded civilization and probably before. Consider the severe wounds and amputations that have always accompanied warfare. Whether one reads the *Iliad* and the *Odyssey*, accounts of Alexander the Great's conquests, Middle Eastern classics such as *Gilgamesh*, or the records of the Aztecs or early Chinese dynasties, one finds that warriors fought, bled, were treated, and lived. There is no indication from these early records that gangrene, sepsis, and other infections killed more warriors than did battlefield wounds, as has occurred in most modern wars. Why not?

One clue may be found in the Smith Papyrus of 1700 B.C. and the Ebers Papyrus of 1500 B.C. Both describe packing very severe wounds and burns with a combination of coagulated milk and honey kept in place by a muslin bandage. This combination or a similar mixture has been used by peoples as diverse as the Romans, eastern African tribes, American Indians, and rural Southerners in the United States. The holy Koran of Islam also recognized the therapeutic value of honey: "Thy Lord has inspired the Bees, / to build their hives in hills / on trees and in man's habitations, / From within their bodies comes / a drink of varying colours, / wherein is healing for mankind." Honey is also a very common ingredient in the traditional Chinese pharmaco-poeia, appearing in treatments for wounds and burns from the earliest to the most modern records. During World War II, for example, people in Shanghai used a honey and lard mixture for treating ulcers and small wounds. Medical practitioners claimed that the results were "excellent." Isak Dinesen, author of *Out of Africa,* also found honey very effective for burns suffered by her native helpers in Kenya.

In Mexico the ancient Aztecs treated many wounds with salted honey. They also discovered a concoction of concentrated maguey sap that acted in a similar way. The maguey plant, a species of agave, has very high concentrations of sugars that form a syrup upon evaporation. Its extracts have been shown to have potent antimicrobial activity. Similarly, generations of New Englanders have recommended honey for the treatment of burns. Indeed, honey, sugar, and plant preparations containing high proportions of sugar appear so often in the materia medica of the past that one might think the sweet stuff some magic potion.

Nonsense? Well, by the mid-1970s scattered medical reports from around the world were beginning to suggest wide-ranging uses for sugar pastes and honey. In 1966 a nurse at the Frenchay Hospital in Bristol, England, reported that two men suffering from bedsores and infected amputations resistant to standard treatments were successfully healed using honey. She had gotten the idea from an article in a popular magazine! Around the same time Arab and Ukrainian physicians reported that honey was useful for treating ear, nose, and throat infections. Russian physicians employed honey to treat skin infections, infections of the urethra, and infections of the eye. German doctors found that a combination of honey mixed with the anesthetic procaine was an effective treatment for herpes zoster, or shingles.

In addition, some British doctors used honey to enhance healing following operations for cancers of the vulva; in India doctors used it to treat skin ulcers and leprosy; and, in New Zealand and Australia, to treat vaginal and abdominal infections and tropical ulcers. Russian and German surgeons even found that honey solutions preserved donor tissues such as blood vessels, bones, and corneas from infection and decay between excision and transplantation into a recipient. They called the process "melitization," from *mel,* the Latin word for honey. By the end of the 1970s the use of honey was common enough that a review of standard wound dressings used by British hospitals included "castor oil and honey."

Despite the growing grass-roots use of honey and sugar pastes in medical practice, controlled clinical testing of their efficacy only began in 1976. In that year two physicians working on separate continents decided independently to find out just how much truth there was to a practice still very much based on hearsay. Both regularly treated patients with incurable bedsores, burn-related infections, and other trauma-related injuries. Both were told, by nurses who had heard about the treatment from older relatives, that sugar healed difficult wounds. Faced with recalcitrant infections on a daily basis, each physician resolved to test sugar pastes scientifically. There was nothing to lose but ignorance.

Dr. Leon Herszage, an Argentinian surgeon working at the Torcuato de Alvear Hospital in Buenos Aires, was the first to publish his results. In 1980 he reported that over the course of the previous four years he had applied sterilized granulated sugar to the surgical wounds of 120 patients and had achieved a cure rate of over 99 percent. Dr. Richard Knutson, a Greenville, Mississippi, orthopedic surgeon, worked with patients in a trauma clinic of the Delta Orthopedic Center, where he treated burns, ulcers, lacerations, gunshot wounds, and amputations. His five-year study of 605 patients treated with sugar-iodine pastes, published in 1981, showed that 98 percent experienced complete healing. He has since treated several thousand patients, with a nearly 99 percent success rate. These figures compare to 94 percent for patients in the same clinics with the same types of injuries and infections who were treated with the more usual antiseptics and antibiotics. The sugar treatment worked better.

The cure rate was only the beginning of the story. Even more phenomenal was the speed of healing in sugar-treated patients. Even wounds that had become infected during the course of standard treatments or that could not be controlled by them would, after a few days of sugar treatment, become sterile and begin to heal. Between 1976 and 1980, the average number of hospital visits required per wound among Knutson's patients dropped from nearly fifty to ten. Whereas 40 percent of his trauma patients who did not receive sugar treatments required skin grafts, not one of the patients treated with sugar ointments did. Herszage reported similarly spectacular results. In other words, in large-scale, clinically controlled trials, Herszage and Knutson both rediscovered what Martín had learned by word of mouth and trial and error in poverty-stricken Ajoya: sugar was not only more effective than standard treatments, but more economical in terms of length, complication, and cost of care.

In some cases sugar-based therapies have even worked medical miracles. Dr. Harvey Gordon and his colleagues at the Northwick Park Hospital and Clinical Research Centre in Harrow, England, had one patient with enormous abscesses in each buttock that were so debilitating the man could not walk and so painful that changing bandages required general anesthesia. No standard treatment brought about any improvement. In desperation the doctors turned to sugar. After packing the patient's abscesses with a paste of sugar and hydrogen peroxide for three days, anesthesia was no longer required, and the patient could get up and walk about for the first time in months. His wounds were completely healed within six weeks. These physicians reported equally striking success with another patient, who had suffered for six months with abscesses on his neck. This patient, too, was completely healed within six weeks. Similar recoveries have since been reported, by physicians on every continent, for patients suffering from ulcerations associated with sickle cell anemia, diabetes, and immune dysfunction.

More surprisingly, surgeons Jean Louis Trouillet, Jean Chastre, and their colleagues at Bichat Hospital in Paris have reported that sugar works not only on external infections but on localized internal ones as well. Like many other heart surgeons, they had a number of patients whose chest wounds became chronically infected following open-heart surgery. When standard antiseptic and antibiotic approaches failed, Trouillet and Chastre packed the open chest cavity around the heart with ordinary sugar, replacing the paste daily by means of a simple suction-tube apparatus. The surgical wounds became sterile within a week on average, fevers associated with infection disappeared within a few days, and the number of patients who died of infection dropped precipitously. As Herszage and Knutson had found, the healing time was hastened dramatically. Average hospital stays following the start of treatment were fifty-four days for patients treated with sugar as opposed to eighty-five days for those treated by conventional methods. Moreover, most patients found the sugar dressing changes to be nearly painless, and little or no anesthetic or analgesic had to be administered, again in distinct contrast to the patients treated according to the usual regimen. Trouillet and Chastre gave new meaning to the words "My wounded heart yearns for your sweet touch."

Severe burns also respond well to sugar and honey treatment. Many of Knutson's patients had suffered burns, and his observations of healing were amply confirmed by an Indian physician, Dr. M. Subrahmanyam. Dr. Subrahmanyam reported in a series of articles in British surgical journals that honey dressings outperformed much more common burn treatments such as silver sulfadiazine gauze dressings and OpSite, a polyurethane film impregnated with antiseptics. Equally glowing recommendations for honey have come from physicians treating burns in North Africa. Surgeons in Asia and Africa are, in fact, eagerly packing honey into an ever-widening variety of wounds. Studies in India have shown that, for cesarean sections, applying honey and taping the incision is more effective and less painful than using traditional dressings and suturing the incision. Honey has also been used for wound care in Indian veterinary practices.

Perhaps the most striking observation of all is that honey may be useful for treating stomach ulcers. Until recently stomach ulcers were thought to be caused by stress and the overproduction of acids, which ate away the lining of the stomach. In Western medicine ulcers have, in consequence, been treated with acid-reducing medications. However, it is now believed that most stomach ulcers are caused by a bacterium, *Helicobacter pylori,* which can effectively be treated with various combinations of antibiotics. We can now conjecture why physicians in the Arabic world, the Caucasus, and Russia have for centuries treated stomach ulcers successfully with honey. In concentrated doses taken orally, honey does have sufficient antibacterial power to kill *Helicobacter.* Thus yet another aspect of honey folklore seems likely to prove true. And in this instance, stomach ulcer patients who are allergic to standard antibiotics may find honey to be a godsend.

The success of sugar and honey treatments has led to an interest in discovering how they exert their curative powers. Sugars have been used to preserve food for hundreds and probably thousands of years, so their antimicrobial properties have been known in a practical way for a very long time. By the mid-1950s a number of bacteriologists demonstrated that honey has profound antibacterial and antifungal effects against human pathogens as well. For example, Dr. W. G. Sackett, a bacteriologist at the Colorado Agriculture College in Fort Collins, tested the antibacterial activity of honey on typhoid, pneumococci, streptococci, dysentery, and many other bacteria. Without exception, all were killed within a few days of exposure to honey, and most within a few hours. A Turkish bacteriologist, N. Ulker, showed that honey could also kill mycobacteria, the germs responsible for tuberculosis and leprosy. And Guido Majno, while writing *The Healing Hand,* a classic history of ancient wound care, actually recreated a number of honey pastes and found that they were excellent antiseptics that quickly killed staphylococci and *Escherichia coli.* More recent studies have confirmed these findings and extended them to other contaminants of surgical wounds as well as many fungi.

The mechanism by which sugars, either in pure form or in honey, exert their antibiotic effects is incompletely understood. On the one hand, sugar appears to stimulate phagocytosis, the process by which white blood cells ingest and destroy germs. On the other hand, they also appear to protect tissues from infection in the same way that they preserve jellies, jams, and conserves from bacteria and fungi. As the Mexican healer Martín pointed out to Singer, the high concentration of sugar creates such high osmotic pressure that germs cannot survive. To understand osmotic pressure you have to appreciate that sugars and salts absorb water. All cells use this osmotic effect to regulate their water content. If, however, there is suddenly more sugar or salt outside the cell than inside, the water will be pulled out of it, causing cell death. This can work to medical advantage, since disease-causing microbes, which are also cells, shrivel up and die in a paste of sugar or honey.

You might expect that body cells in contact with high concentrations of sugars or salts would also shrivel and die, but that is not the case. The body's tissue cells are in communication with one another and with the circulatory and lymph systems. Cells that are part of a larger system compensate for detrimental osmotic pressures by drawing water continuously from the rest of the body. At the same time, body cells begin metabolizing the sugars, drawing them away from the wound for use by the body. Only damaged cells or single cells such as germs that are not part of a body system are actually threatened by the presence of sugars. The destruction of damaged body cells due to high sugar concentrations may, in fact, be an additional benefit of sugar-based therapies, since dead tissue provides a breeding ground for many types of bacteria, including those associated with bedsores and gangrene. Thus sugar-based treatments may create an effective and painless form of debridement that eliminates dead tissue while sterilizing the wound.

Interestingly enough, honey is a more effective antifungal and antibacterial agent than is sugar, suggesting that honey contains antimicrobial ingredients. Some of these have been identified. Most honeys contain relatively high levels of hydrogen peroxide, a highly reactive chemical that is produced as a natural part of the body's immune response to pathogens. Hydrogen peroxide is, in fact, widely sold by drugstores as an antiseptic. (Recall that

Gordon and his colleagues at Harrow successfully tested a sugar and hydrogen-peroxide combination.) The higher the hydrogen-peroxide content of the honey, the more effective it is in killing germs. Peroxides also stimulate white blood cells called macrophages, which initiate the overall immune response to infection.

In addition to peroxides, honeys contain other active ingredients such as formic acid, which acts in a similar way to hydrogen peroxide. And most honeys contain significant amounts of vitamins, including vitamin C, and trace amounts of a wide range of minerals, including iron, copper, manganese, calcium, potassium, sodium, phosphorus, and magnesium. All of these components may increase its osmotic pressure, and all are essential for the activation and repair of body cells. These substances probably add to honey's wound-healing effects. Finally, it is possible that honey contains growth factors, which are components of almost all body secretions and have been found to stimulate wound healing.

Reports that sugar and honey decrease the need for skin grafts and plastic surgery are also beginning to make sense in light of the most recent medical research. Mark Ferguson of the University of Manchester, England, has discovered that certain sugars can retard the regrowth of collagen, the fibrous protein that makes up connective tissue and that is overproduced to form scar tissue. By making experimental incisions in his own arms, he has shown that specific sugars can largely prevent scarring. "The treated wound is not completely invisible," he writes, "but it is much, much less noticeable than the untreated one." If clinical studies verify Ferguson's laboratory findings, and if these sugars are approved by the U.S. Food and Drug Administration for general use, this discovery could be very good news for those who suffer from the excessive formation of scar tissue, or keloids. In the meantime, you may have to make do with honey and sugar pastes, if you can convince your physician to use them!

All in all, then, sugar and honey are very versatile medicines. Does that mean that apiaries may one day be owned by pharmaceutical companies? It is not beyond imagination. But more likely, scientists will exploit the healing properties of honeys and sugars by creating artificial mixtures of sugars, hydrogen peroxide, vitamins, minerals, salts, and perhaps even growth factors. In the meantime, physicians like Knutson and healers like Martín use a mixture of Betadine with specially prepared, sterilized, unadulterated sugar. Knutson has gone so far as to suggest that mixing ordinary table sugar or honey into some sterile butter or margarine will produce a home remedy for cuts and scrapes that is "just as effective and comforting as anything available on the market." It is important to note, however, that most commercially available sugar is not sterile and contains calcium chloride, flour, or other materials to prevent caking. Moreover, some honeys have been reported to have low levels of the bacteria that cause botulism or other toxins that can be harmful to infants and people with preexisting medical problems. Thus most medical professionals do not recommend home use of commercially available sugars and honeys.

The very possibility that sugar and honey can be used (and misused) at home without medical supervision may explain not only the survival of this therapy as folk medicine but also the strong medical resistance it has met with in some quarters. Martín knew that his methods "are not approved by the medical societies." Similarly Knutson has said, "When I first started to publicize this [sugar] treatment, all the doctors threw a lot of stones at me." And some "stone throwing" continues, despite a steady accumulation of evidence. A recent article in *Time* magazine described the medical community's "cold shoulder for a burn 'cure'" developed in China called Moist Burn Ointment. The "inventor" of the ointment, Dr. Xu Rong Xiang, claims that the ointment reduces pain on contact, minimizes scarring, and cuts healing time by up to a third. Most American specialists who have reviewed the Chinese results remain "skeptical." Only a few, such as physicians at the National Burn Foundation, based in New Jersey, are taking Moist Burn Ointment seriously. As might have been expected, a major component of the ointment is, once again, honey. And Xu Rong Xiang comes from a family of natural healers.

Herein, we suspect, lies the crux of the matter. Modern societies have come to equate medical knowledge with formalized university training. It is hard for most of us to believe that an unaccredited healer such as Martín, or even a doctor trained outside the hallowed halls of Western medicine such as Dr. Xiang, might be able to cure conditions that the best-trained Harvard Medical School graduate despairs of treating. But formal academic systems are only one of many ways in which knowledge is discovered, accumulated, and transmitted. Folk cultures may also spontaneously and in isolation from one another develop efficacious medicines and pass them down from generation to generation.

Thus when Singer asked Martín, "Where did you learn this technique?" his question had profound implications that went far beyond the issue of sugar treatments. And Martin seems to have realized these implications: "I learned it here and there, but mostly by treating people every day, and every day you learn something. It's a lie, whoever says, 'I know how to do it.' There's always something else to learn. Every day one has to learn by trying different methods of how to cure the people more actively. You can learn things in hospitals, schools, everywhere, but the best school is practice." And sometimes, that school teaches, the best treatment is sweet.

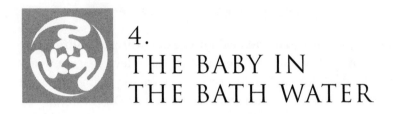

4.
THE BABY IN
THE BATH WATER

*One of the intriguing facets of medical progress is
our continuing rediscovery of the past, a fascinating
example of which is the recent widespread
application of the ancient therapeutic modality of
water immersion.*

— Murray Epstein, M.D., 1992

FOR AS LONG as anyone could remember,
sick people had come from miles around to
soak in the temperate spring that bubbled up from the ground
near the small village of Buxton in Derbyshire, England. By the
late 1600s a bath had been constructed to hold the water and a
room built over it to keep the air warm and provide some measure
of protection and privacy. Men and women bathed separately,
sitting up to their necks in water, for two or three hours at a time.
Customarily the sick immersed themselves twice a day for at least
one week and sometimes as many as six weeks. And a great many
of them were cured of their ailments.

Accounts of the healing waters were passed by word of
mouth. Written affidavits were collected by the keeper of the bath.
Eventually these found their way into print. Caleb Pott, a school-
master suffering from gout, "came thither on his Crutches, and
went away very well, and testify'd this under his hand, 1689." Mr.
Stephen Kaye, rector, faithfully attended the baths for four years in
a row and was "cured of the Gravel in the Kidneys, which tortur'd
him for several Years: And also of the Gout, to which he was

44

subject." Edmund Horncastle used the bath and "recover'd of his Lameness and Pains, and went away without his Crutches." In 1691 Mr. Fauler was cured of "a Rheumatism mixt with the Dropsie and Scurvy." And after a two-week course of the waters, a gentleman from York recovered from a relapse of the "cold Palsey."

Oral and written testimonies such as these, gathered over hundreds of years, buoyed people up in the past. They believed that bathing in the waters of Buxton was just the right medicine for a host of acute and chronic conditions, including rickets, fever, itching, ringworm, apoplexy, palsy, melancholy, jaundice, dropsy, rheumatism, gout, kidney stones, ulcers, colic, dysentery, gonorrhea, infertility, and inflammation of the liver. Nor were the springs of Buxton the only waters believed to confer relief from such diseases. The mineral springs of Bath were also said to cure constipation, colic, gout, infertility, and paralysis.

Across the Channel in Europe hundreds of mineral springs were exploited for similar purposes. Michelangelo "tried" the waters at Fiuggi in 1559 to relieve his suffering from kidney stones. The French essayist Michel de Montaigne in 1580 took to the waters of Plombières-les-Bains in France, Baden in Switzerland, and Bagni di Lucca in Italy, in the hopes that one or all would be, as one doctor assured him, "marvellously good for liver complaints . . . and for the stone and colic as well." And the English writer Tobias Smollett, though he satirized medical bathing at Bath in many of his novels, resorted to the waters of Aix-les-Bains in France to cure an "ugly scorbutic tetter," or ulcer, that had robbed him of the use of his right hand. Therapeutic pilgrimages such as these were common among the rich and, by the eighteenth and nineteenth centuries, taking the waters was the fashionable thing to do, whether or not you were sick. Even the poor had their turn in the pools, some of which were set aside specifically for charity patients. Mineral-spring baths had few rivals as one of the most popular curative agents in the history of medicine.

The use of certain springs dates back thousands of years. Evidence from the Swiss Alps and from the Russian shores of the Black Sea suggests that prehistoric people pooled the waters of mineral springs in order to bathe. In England legend has it that around 860 B.C. a royal leper named Bladud cured himself by plunging into a steaming swamp by the Avon River, thus establishing a therapeutic use for the springs later known as Bath. The Mayan people left archaeological evidence of their use of mineral springs, as did the ancient Greeks and Romans and the Japanese, who used hot springs both to heat and to heal their bodies.

Written records of ancient medicinal uses of mineral-spring bathing also exist. The Romans particularly prescribed such baths for paralysis, sciatica, skin complaints such as psoriasis, rheumatic disorders, gout, as well as other chronic complaints that we now associate with liver and kidney failure, such as jaundice and edema. A similar emphasis can be found in medical texts from other cultures. From the eighth to the sixteenth centuries, Chinese physicians prescribed mineral-spring bathing for cramps, convulsions, rheumatism, paralysis, skin complaints, and syphilitic ulcers. Modern therapeutic indications for bathing in mineral springs in India, which are said to reflect local customs dating back 2500 years, also include skin diseases, rheumatism, paralysis, and metabolic disorders. The ancient Hindus are thought to have practiced a formal therapeutic use of mineral waters known as *jalachikitsa*. Such bathing was said not only to clean the skin but to purify the blood, improve eyesight, and increase appetite and seminal secretions.

Of course, in many religious cultures — the Egyptian, Islamic, Hindu, Chinese, Hebrew, Greek, Roman, and Christian — bathing also had spiritual meaning. Rituals of immersion in water symbolized religious purification in many cases; in other instances immersion was hygienic, a purification of the hair and skin. More often than not, the spiritual and the physical were blended in perceptions of medicinal cleansing. At Bath the story of the leper's miraculous cure inspired such awe that the waters were believed to represent the healing powers of Celtic and, later, Roman gods. The Romans, in fact, routinely built shrines as well as baths at their mineral springs. And at Lourdes, France, where the "miraculous" power of the springs to heal the crippled and sick was discovered by religious vision, bathing and prayer have always gone hand in hand.

Because of religious associations, hygienic results, and "miracle" cures, bathing in any water has deep significance. Language itself reflects the origins of bathing at mineral springs first discovered millennia ago. In English we take a "bath," recalling the famous springs of Bath, England. The same is true of the French word *bain*, the Italian *bagni*, and the German *bad*, all of which referred originally to mineral springs rather than the humble household bath. Moreover, today when we engage in more public, therapeutic bathing, we go to a health resort or spa, recalling the famous Espa (meaning "fountain") springs of Spa, Belgium, discovered by an ironmonger in the early 1300s.

Thus in language, ritual, and daily hygiene, we mark our kinship to the many people who took themselves to Spa, Bath, Buxton, Plombières, Lourdes, and Baden. But few of us today take baths to cure paralysis, ease gout or rheumatism, soothe an ulcer, or treat ailments of the liver or the heart. Bathing for medicinal purposes went out with horse-drawn carriages, a quaint but outmoded practice of people less sophisticated than ourselves. The question we must pose is whether medicinal bathing was also an effective technology bypassed by subsequent developments or whether it was a form of quackery that resulted in mass delusion. Were all the doctors who presided at mineral springs taking advantage of the sick people who flocked there? Were all the people who swore by their bathing regimens simply deceived? Or was the proverbial baby tossed out with the bath water when balneotherapy, as it is called, was finally discarded by the medical profession?

Around 1983 Drs. J. P. O'Hare, Audrey Heywood, and their colleagues at the Royal Infirmary in Bristol, England, decided to try to answer these questions. Experts in the physiological effects of head-out immersion (sitting in water up to the neck), the team decided to test the physiological effects of an actual mineral-spring bath. In what Harold Conn, a professor of internal medicine at Yale, has called a "delicious" episode, O'Hare, Heywood, and the rest of the team approached the Bath City Council for permission to use water from one of the hot-spring baths. These baths, along with all other therapeutic spas in Great Britain, had been closed a number of years previously as a cost-cutting measure, and public funds for their medicinal use had been withdrawn. Though unable to use the baths on site, O'Hare obtained permission to cart some of the spa water to Bristol.

The research quickly became an adventure with distinct overtones of a Monty Python comedy. O'Hare's team pumped five hundred gallons of Bath mineral water into a "bowser," or water tank on wheels, and hauled it to the Bristol Royal Infirmary by taxi. Once there the scientists tried pumping the water straight from the tank in the parking lot to the immersion laboratory five floors above ground. In a parody of scientific writing, they reported that, unfortunately, "pump failure supervened," and "attempts at resuscitation failed." Not to be deterred, however, a team of "healthy volunteers" worked up a good sweat by carrying the five hundred gallons of mineral water into the building by hand. By this time clearly aware of the comic nature of their enterprise, the team even made a photographic record of the project's staggering steps.

Once the experimental baths were filled, O'Hare and his colleagues reenacted a spa "cure" on eight unidentified subjects (evidence strongly suggests that they were the eight team members themselves). Like patients at Bath in the eighteenth century, each volunteer drank water upon waking and spent the morning immersed up to the neck in a warm (35 degrees centigrade) mineral-water bath. Periodically the unimmersed researchers drew blood, collected urine output, and monitored the volunteers' blood flow and heart functions.

As the measurements accumulated, O'Hare, Heywood, and the others recognized their similarity to experimental data they and other investigators had gathered over the previous decade for quite other reasons. One of the earliest studies on record of the physiological effects of prolonged head-out bathing was performed by the American physiologist H. C. Bazett around 1920. Bazett observed that a marked diuresis, or increased urinary excretion, was one of the most characteristic effects of such baths on healthy men. Further study demonstrated that whether the water was cold, tepid, or warm made no difference in this effect, but full immersion of the trunk of the body did. Partial immersion of the limbs alone, or even the shallow immersion of a home bathtub, did not cause increased urination. Sitting up to the neck in a pool for a few hours, however, clearly increased the excretion of water, salts, and urea, the chief components of urine.

Bazett's observations, made at a time when spas were going out of fashion, were largely ignored. Interest in immersion studies was reawakened in a quite unexpected quarter, however, when Americans decided to send men into outer space during the late 1950s and '60s. Asked to predict how the astronauts would respond to the weightlessness of zero gravity, physiologists realized they did not know. What they did know, however, was that due to the buoyancy of bodies in dense liquids, water immersion provided a ready-made experimental analogue on earth to zero gravity. In consequence, astronauts and other volunteers spent hours, sometimes days, in tanks of water simulating the physiological effects of weightlessness. And just as Bazett would have predicted, they urinated like crazy, excreted tremendous amounts of salt and urea, and got very, very thirsty.

The scientists conducting these studies were gratified to find that the astronauts in orbital space flights experienced the same effects and were adequately prepared to deal with them. Equally gratifying was the resurgence of interest in immersion as a research tool for studying how the body regulates its salts and fluids. "In the process," wrote Murray Epstein of the University of Miami Medical School and one of the leaders of immersion research, "[medical scientists] have rediscovered some of the historically neglected benefits of immersion and applied them to modern investigations of physiology and the pathophysiology of many disease states."

Epstein and others recognized the applications of their research to treating disease, but oddly enough, none of them explicitly connected the effects of head-out immersion to the historical

uses of mineral-spring baths. This was the task of O'Hare, Heywood, and their team. Not surprisingly, they found that their eight
volunteers also urinated heavily and became thirsty. But being
true scientists, they took nothing for granted. When they were
done with the Bath water, they poured all five hundred gallons of
it down the drain and repeated the regimen on the same eight
volunteers using warm Bristol tap water. To quote the laconic
conclusion of their unusual report: "No significant differences
were observed." Water from Bath is just bath water, at least as far as
its physical effects on an immersed individual. All that work for
such a mundane answer.

Actually, the data that the team collected is really quite interesting, not because it was unforeseen but because it verified that
spa bathing had significant effects on the body's excretory processes and that these effects were the same as expected from immersion in any water. The true novelty of the O'Hare study is that
it was the first to link spa therapies with the known physiological
effects of bathing and conclude that such therapies in the past
may therefore have had true medicinal value.

The sort of therapeutic value it had largely depended upon
the physiological effects of water immersion, which went beyond
excretory functions. Because all of the body's systems are integrated, the excretion of water, salt, and urea necessarily affects
many other functions as well, especially regulation of blood volume and pressure. Head-out immersion creates greater pressure
on the lower body relative to the upper body. Blood is therefore
compressed out of the limbs and into the trunk, like toothpaste in
a tube squeezed from the bottom up. Volume receptors in the
trunk sense the rise in blood volume and elicit compensatory
mechanisms, such as urination, to return the volume to normal by
reducing the amount of water in the blood. At the same time,
because water is supporting the body, the effects of gravity are
lessened, and blood pressure drops. What this means therapeutically is that people in the past who had hypertension (high blood
pressure), circulatory problems, or one of the many diseases in

which fluid is retained probably benefited from prolonged bathing in spa waters.

During the 1970s, recognition that immersion affects control of blood volume led Murray Epstein and other investigators, including Daniel Bichet of the University of Colorado Health Sciences Center, to use it as a research tool in the study of specific diseases characterized by blood-volume imbalances. These include liver, kidney, and heart ailments resulting in excessive fluid retention. Cirrhosis of the liver results in retention of salt, decreased urination, and the consequent buildup of fluid (as much as twenty-eight liters!) in the tissues of the abdomen, a condition known as ascites. Dropsy — what we today call edema — is most often associated with nephrotic syndrome (a degeneration of the kidneys) and congestive heart failure, both of which can cause very noticeable swelling of the limbs due to fluid retention. (If you ever noticed that Great-Grandma's ankles looked twice as fat as her shoes, she probably had some form of dropsy.) Without intervention, both edema and ascites can become progressively worse, because the body "misinterprets" what is going on. Buildup of fluid in tissues can result in decreased blood volume, which the body's sensors read as a signal to increase fluid retention. For reasons that are still not fully understood, however, in disease states the additional fluid moves inappropriately into body tissues rather than remaining in the blood. A vicious cycle that can lead to death begins.

Most modern cases of liver disease complicated by ascites can be satisfactorily treated with drugs that increase urination. But patients with refractory ascites, unresponsive to conventional treatment, pose a special problem. Some physicians wondered if water immersion could be manipulated clinically; in other words, could the diuresis observed in research subjects with ascites — as modest as it was — be used to control or cure the condition? In one case reported in 1987, a middle-aged tax inspector with ascites failed to respond to drug therapy. Over the course of some ten days he took three prolonged up-to-the-neck baths along with drug therapy and experienced the complete elimination of his ascites. The physicians responsible for his treatment — and they included the Dr. O'Hare who tested the mineral waters of Bath — suggested that "the use of . . . diuretics combined with water immersion is a safe and effective method of treating those cirrhotics with ascites who fail to respond to conventional treatment." Subsequently, physicians in Germany, Poland, and the former Czechoslovakia repeated the clinical combination of diuretics and water immersion with equally beneficial results.

Early in the 1980s immersion was also seriously considered as a medical therapy for patients suffering from a range of kidney diseases. Experimental research by two different groups indicated that nephrotic patients experienced much the same physical effects from immersion as the normal or cirrhotic bather. Some patients lost up to two kilograms of fluid in the form of sweat as well as urine, which brought about an obvious diminution of edema. Even those who experienced no major fluid loss felt subjective relief from swollen ankles. The researchers concluded that prolonged bathing was not only simple and therapeutically promising but also psychologically beneficial. With some success physicians have even turned to water immersion in the attempt to reverse hepatorenal syndrome, a kind of kidney failure due to liver disease that is almost always fatal.

Late-pregnancy toxemia has also been treated with bathing. In this condition the pregnant woman experiences a buildup of body fluids at the expense of blood volume. Salt is retained, and blood pressure often rises dangerously. Toxemia is associated with retarded fetal growth and dramatically increased risk of death to both the mother and the baby. As with other forms of fluid retention, various diuretic drugs can be useful, but their effects on the fetus are not well established. Physical methods of shifting fluids from the limbs into the central body cavity to induce urination and excretion of salt have therefore been attempted, including lower-body pressure suits and head-out immersion. Only bathing was found to be successful in reversing the problems associated with toxemia.

High blood pressure that is resistant to drug therapy has also been treated with head-out immersion. The greatest strides in this area have been made by the Russians as an offshoot of their use of immersion to simulate zero-gravity effects for their space program. They invented a "dry immersion technique" in which the body is protected from contact with water by a thin plastic sheet, making much longer periods of "immersion" possible. Recently, this sort of "bathing" has been used to treat patients suffering from essential hypertension.

These modern studies tell us that for certain diseases involving fluid retention deep-water immersion was in the past — and still is today — an effective physical medicine. The surprising thing is that other diseases, some of which no longer plague us, may also have responded to bathing. Here we rejoin Audrey Heywood, a member of O'Hare's Bath water team, who reasoned that if urinary excretion of salts benefited conditions such as hypertension, the excretion of other substances may have effectively treated other diseases. She began by delving into the records maintained at the Bath Hospital since the early eighteenth century to see what physicians in the past had claimed to cure. She quickly found that one form of paralysis in particular, known as *colica pictonum,* apparently responded well to spa therapy.

Unheard of today, *colica pictonum* was characterized by a short episode of severe abdominal colic (paroxysms of pain), followed by a permanent palsy, or loss of sensation and control, in the hands or arms. Of the paralytic patients treated at Bath, 7 percent suffered from this condition, and most were considered incurable by other doctors using other methods. According to hospital records, resident physicians believed that bathing in Bath waters completely cured almost half of these *colica pictonum* patients and obviously benefited nearly all. Heywood's next question was why spa therapy should have served these patients so well. She found her clue in the cause of the disease.

In 1768 it was recognized that a number of palsies initially thought to be distinct from one another and from *colica pictonum* were, in fact, all caused by chronic lead poisoning. Since Roman times lead poisoning had been common in Europe, due to the use of the metal in water pipes, earthenware, cooking pots, pewter plates and tankards, cosmetics, hair dyes, and medicines. Lead absorbed through the mucous membranes or skin preferentially concentrates in the nerves, leading to such symptoms as uncontrollable shaking, loss of sensation, weakness in the limbs, numbness, deafness, impotence, memory loss, and confusion. Many cases of colic, paralysis, and abnormal mental behavior throughout the ages were therefore probably caused by lead poisoning in one form or another; in the eighteenth century it was often the result of drinking rum and other liquors fermented in lead stills.

Once Heywood knew that *colica pictonum* was caused by lead poisoning, everything else fell into place. First of all, she knew that one of the substances excreted during immersion is calcium. Second, she knew that ingested lead replaces calcium in many physiological systems. Perhaps, she hypothesized, bathing had the same effect on lead in the body as it has on calcium. This led to another experiment. A new immersion study was undertaken in which the amount of lead excreted in urine was measured during three-hour baths in warm water up to the neck. The results confirmed that excretion of lead, as of sodium and calcium, does increase during bathing. Although the amount of lead excreted in one three-hour bath is small, several such baths per week over some twenty-four weeks — typical for a cure at Bath in the eighteenth century — would have significantly reduced the amount of lead in the body. Drinking the waters, an additional mode of therapy at most bathing sites, would also have increased the amount of urine produced and therefore the amount of lead excreted. As long as additional ingestion of lead was avoided, as was likely to be the case for patients following the regimen of eating and drinking recommended by spa physicians, the paralysis of *colica pictonum* could be completely reversed, just as the Bath records indicated.

Heywood went on to conjecture that this simple internal cleansing of the body by repeated bathing may have brought relief from other symptoms of lead poisoning as well, such as lassitude, headaches, and infertility, all of which were common complaints among people attending European spas in the past. Perhaps most striking is the connection between lead poisoning and gout, a condition in which excess uric acid crystals are deposited in the joints of the big toe, the ankle, and the knee, causing protuberant swelling and acute attacks of pain. Today we understand gout to be primarily an inherited disorder, resulting from the inability to metabolize or break down an excretory product called uric acid. Small, regular doses of lead can also induce gout in susceptible people.

In the eighteenth century this sort of gout appears to have reached epidemic proportions among wealthy English land-owners and merchants with an excessive fondness for port contaminated with lead from storage in lead-lined casks or from contact with leaded pewter. Indeed, the image of the corpulent, well-to-do man, his foot wrapped in bandages, was indelibly etched in satirical scenes of spa towns like Bath. Deep-water bathing probably reversed cases of lead-induced gout by increasing the excretion of the metabolic poison. Inherited forms of gout, usually associated with an inability to urinate copiously, may not have responded as well to immersion. However, if the sufferer also drank large amounts of water, as was recommended, even inherited gout may have been somewhat alleviated, since any induced urination would also mean the excretion of uric acid. Spa therapies were certainly prescribed for gouty patients through the 1930s in the United States and continue to be used today in conjunction with drug therapy in France, Germany, Italy, Poland, and Russia.

In premodern times the term "gout" actually referred to any rheumatic inflammatory disease: rheumatoid arthritis, rheumatic fever, inherited gout, lead-associated gout, and so forth. Well aware of this, Heywood, O'Hare, and their associates had already tried head-out immersion in the treatment of rheumatoid arthritis, a chronic and progressive inflammation, swelling, and stiffening of the joints. In 1984 they immersed seven rheumatic patients and, sure enough, found that as urination increased, joint swelling decreased. "These physiological changes could be important in modifying disease processes in patients using water immersion as a therapy," they concluded. In fact, in a number of countries, including Israel and Japan, mineral-spring bathing has long been prescribed for the treatment of rheumatic complaints, including rheumatoid arthritis and a related problem called ankylosing spondylitis (arthritis of the spine). In some of these instances, the healing effects of increased circulation due to the warmth of the water cannot be separated from the benefits of greater fluid excretion. Researchers have not yet adequately appraised the therapeutic mechanisms, but frankly the patients don't care. They feel better, and that's what counts for them.

In sum, mineral-spring bathing was no mass delusion of yesteryear, but was, rather, a historically viable medical therapy. It may have been an overstatement for an eighteenth-century postcard to proclaim Bath waters "the Most Sovereign Restorative," but it wasn't too far off in claiming that the waters were "Wonderful and *most* EXCELLENT agaynst all *diseases* of the body proceeding of a MOIST CAUSE as Rhumes, Agues, Lethargies, *Apoplexies,* The Scratch, *Inflammation of the Fits,* hectic flushes, Pockes, deafness, *forgetfulness,* shakings and WEAKNESS of any Member — Approved by authoritie, confirmed by Reason and daily tried by experience." Modern research confirms that deep-water bathing is good for cirrhosis of the liver with ascites, kidney disease with edema, lead-induced paralysis of the arms, lead-induced gout, rheumatoid arthritis, and simple high blood pressure.

We cannot leave the subject of immersion without some caveats, however. Occasionally people were harmed by their spa regimens. Renaissance physicians recognized that certain mineral or hot baths could provoke a range of side effects, such as headaches, convulsions, copious sweat, fever, vomiting, even death, and warned against their excessive use. Similar injunctions were issued by English physicians into the early nineteenth century. It may be that some of these adverse effects were due to ingestion of the mineral waters or to bathing in waters so hot they raised body temperature to dangerous levels. But at least one contraindication concerned the effect of immersion itself. As early as 1535 Paracelsus warned against warm baths in cases of dropsy (edema) due to congestive heart disease. Standard medical practice reiterated that proscription well into the nineteenth century. From modern research we now know that the increase in central blood volume due to water immersion may cause a rapid, pathological heartbeat, or tachycardia, in the already stressed heart, leading to pulmonary congestion and heart failure.

The risks traditionally associated with immersion help to explain why modern American practitioners, although aware of the possible benefits of balneotherapy, have resisted incorporating it into their regular treatment regimens. In addition some physicians think it is too time-consuming and labor intensive, requiring constant supervision of the sick individual, who may fall or faint in the deep tub. Pills, when they work, act faster and better, in the safety of a bed. But other factors have also militated against the modern therapeutic use of immersion. In Great Britain, for instance, the demise of balneotherapy during the past fifty years came about largely because of changes in medical disciplines and professional specialization. Prior to the twentieth century physicians in Britain could specialize by treatment modality, and spa therapies were one such modality. The rise of rheumatology, cardiology, nephrology, and other specialties, however, changed the focus to specialization in one or another organ system. The organ specialists ignored medicinal immersion, and cost-cutting measures by Britain's government-run health-care system forced the closing of the mineral springs. In the United States, as well as in Great Britain, the spa facilities necessary for routine medicinal bathing are now simply lacking.

On the European continent, however, physicians have retained much closer ties to spa therapies. The medical uses of bathing continue to run the gamut of possibilities in terms of water depth, temperature, and length of immersion. In Russia and Central Europe, mineral-water immersion is only one part of a broadly conceived program that includes a variety of water shower, water spray, and gas and mud baths. Virtually every disease under the sun is treated, including gout and paralysis, arthritis, anemic and gynecological conditions, rheumatic fever, cardiovascular disorders, heart defects, and convalescence after gastric surgery. Although the scientific basis for most of these spa therapies has not been confirmed, the medical rediscovery of head-out immersion in water ought to make us just a little less quick to scoff at their persistence. Medicine, as historian Henry Sigerist once wrote, is a field in which the lessons of experience often precede the lessons of science.

And recognizing these lessons raises a new and amazing prospect. This year the National Aeronautics and Space Administration (NASA) began talking with various airlines and travel agencies about the possibility of one day taking people into outer space for recreational purposes. Might the history of medicine repeat itself? Modern researchers rediscovered the efficacy of immersion in the course of studying the physiological effects of weightlessness on earth. Perhaps these same researchers will soon discover ways in which weightlessness can enhance modern therapies for diseases historically treated by bathing in mineral springs. We already know that the physiological effects of zero gravity far surpass those induced by water immersion. In the past our ancestors flocked to earthly springs for spa therapy. In the future our offspring might rocket to the Moon or Mars for a little space therapy. One thing is for sure, if it's out there, they'll find the medical baby in the cosmic bath water!

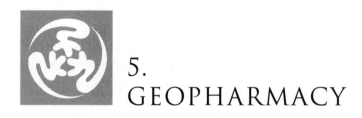

5.
GEOPHARMACY

It may be that the world's oldest medicine is the earth itself.

— Timothy Johns, Ph.D., 1991

I N BADEN, GERMANY, just over four hundred years ago, a condemned criminal faced the hangman. Rather than swing from a rope, however, he made a unique counterproposal to the court. Give me the most deadly poison you have, he said, and I will take it, provided that you give me some terra sigillata at the same time. The dignitaries overseeing the execution agreed.

Terra sigillata, or "earth that has been stamped with a seal," was a clay that had been dug up since time immemorial on only one day of the year, August 6, on the Greek island of Lemnos under the careful oversight in ancient times of the priestesses of Diana and, in the sixteenth century, of secular officials. The clay was mixed with the blood of a sacrificial goat, shaped into lozenges somewhat larger than a thumbnail, stamped with the figure of a goat or some other special seal, and dried. Highly prized, even imitated, the lozenges were believed by various authorities, such as Galen in the second century A.D., to be an antidote to poison. Kings, princes, and popes were known to ingest terra sigillata with their meals as a safeguard against treasonous plots. But did the clay really work?

By 1581, the year in which the criminal trial in Baden took such an unexpected turn, terra sigillata had already been the subject of some of the earliest medical experiments on record. Dogs had been given various poisons along with terra sigillata and had apparently survived. The court in Baden agreed to poison, rather than hang, their prisoner in order to perform a human experiment similar to those tried previously on the dogs.

On the appointed day the prisoner swallowed one and a half drams (about six grams or one teaspoon) of mercuric chloride, a poison that corrodes the mucous membranes and stomach lining, inducing severe nausea, abdominal pain, diarrhea, renal damage, and, in extreme cases, death. The dosage that the prisoner ingested was, according to modern medical studies, three to six times the amount needed to kill an average-size man. The executioners were not leaving anything to chance.

Five minutes after ingesting the mercuric chloride, the prisoner swallowed a dram of terra sigillata in wine. A physician and an apothecary observed the entire course of the treatment. Their somewhat understated report says that the poison "did extremely torment and vexe him: yet in the end the medicine overcame it, whereby the poore wretch was delivered and being restored to his health, was committed to his parents." The medical authorities and the condemned man were both pleased with the outcome. The experiment had been a dirty business, but it had worked.

The purposeful ingestion of clay is by no means confined to the past or to Europe. Half a world away from Greece, on the Indonesian island of Java, a clay preparation called *ampo* is still eaten for nutritional and weight control purposes. *Ampo* is often made from a red-brown clay containing a good deal of iron, but it can be made from clays of other colors as well. Professional preparers called *tukang ampo* oversee a process in which the clay is kneaded into a paste with water, molded into small pencils or round biscuitlike shapes a few centimeters thick, and baked on an iron pan. Once it is done, the clay looks like cooked pork. To enhance its flavor and appeal, it is sometimes molded into the shapes of various animals or salted and spread with vegetable oil before baking.

It is perhaps worth noting that people who have eaten *ampo* say that they have enjoyed it. Its texture has been described as being similar to that of fine chocolate as it melts on the tongue, though with little distinctive flavor, and it has an unusual drying effect on the mouth as it absorbs moisture. Similar descriptions have been given for many other types of "edible" clays from around the world. A few, such as the white clay of Nishapur, Iran; *kartooti*, a claylike mud from Sudan; and lithomarge, or rock marrow, from the southern United States, are even described as tasting sweet.

The thought of eating clay may strike many people in the West as being somewhat, well, dirty. Infants, who will put almost anything in their mouths, are trained very early to avoid ingesting dirt, mud, sand, and rocks. "Dirty," indeed, is a term of opprobrium flung not only at soil but at unclean things in general and, perhaps more significantly, at culturally unacceptable practices such as pornography and foul language. Yet we all unavoidably ingest some dirt during our lives. As Grandma Root used to say, "You gotta eat a peck of dirt before you die!" We don't think she meant that we ought to eat dirt on purpose; that peck was supposed to accumulate by accident: a bit of soil on an unwashed garden tomato, a carrot pulled right out of the ground, given a bit of a rub to get the grit off, then eaten right then and there — that sort of thing. Yet geophagy, or the purposeful eating of earth, be it in the form of clay, dirt, mud, pebbles, rocks, or even pottery and china, is actually far more common than most people would suspect.

The fact is, your neighbors may be eating earth. As a child growing up in Los Angeles, one of us knew an old lady who used to go up the coast every so often to a special spot where she would dig a big lump of clay to bring home and savor at regular intervals. And she was hardly unusual. Surveys have found that as many as 25 percent of children and 50 percent of adult women in rural areas of the American South had eaten dirt or clay at least twice in the previous two weeks. The average amount ingested was about 50 grams, or two ounces, per day. It is, furthermore, a learned behavior. One woman who lives in the Baltimore area admitted that she had been taught to eat clay by her mother and that she had introduced her own daughter to the practice. They regularly went to the Baltimore Brickyard to obtain highly refined red clay. "You never want to eat dirt from the garden — it might have grit in it and set your teeth on edge, but that clay from the brickyard is *so* nice." Potters' clay has also been described by aficionados as being quite fine. We'll even wager that you have purposefully ingested some clay yourself, probably for medicinal purposes but almost surely without knowing it — *terra incognita,* as it were!

We all partake of earthy repasts, and it is essential that we do so. To begin with, almost all of the minerals in our diet come originally from the earth. Plants take up minerals through their roots and incorporate them into their cells. Animals, in turn, eat the plants. Animals can also derive some of their needs from waters containing dissolved minerals. Minerals such as calcium, magnesium, potassium, zinc, iron, selenium, cobalt, and even that modern bugaboo, sodium, are all necessary to life — so important that one could say a dearth of earth is unhealthy. Unfortunately, not everyone in the world derives adequate nutrition from their regular diet. Some malnourished and ill people must turn directly to the earth for sustenance.

If it is difficult to think of clay as food, remember that the salt you sprinkle on your food most likely came from some deposit in the earth. An earthy origin does not necessarily connote uncleanness. In fact, many primitive peoples learned not to drink directly from streams and rivers, but to dig a hole in the mud nearby and allow the hole to fill with water from the bottom up by diffusion through the soil. The result was purified water, not too different from artesian well water that has filtered through hundreds of feet of rock. The earth, in other words, can clean and be clean. To eat the earth itself is not necessarily a dirty act.

Geophagy, though not universal, has been recorded since time immemorial and on every continent. The oldest evidence for it comes from a prehistoric site at Kalambo Falls, Zambia, where the bones of *Homo habilis,* the immediate predecessor of *Homo sapiens,* have been found side by side with a special white clay.

Several facts suggest geophagy: the site predates by tens of thousands of years any known use of clay for making pottery or ornaments; the clay is not found naturally anywhere in the vicinity, suggesting that it was carried there on purpose; and it is of a very special type that has been favored for eating by cultures ever since. Perhaps *Homo habilis* used the clay as a food supplement (analysis showed it to be extremely rich in calcium) or as a detoxicant. Or perhaps they ate it to ward off hunger, to ensure a successful pregnancy, or to cure diseases. All of these possibilities are uses to which similar clays and muds have been put over the millennia.

One of the most common recorded uses of earths is as a food supplement during periods of famine, for in addition to its mineral content, a small amount of clay will remain in the stomach for a long time, dulling the appetite. We can understand the expedient, therefore, of feeding both men and animals *Kieselgur,* or "mountain meal," when famine struck seventeenth-century Germany during the Thirty Years War. Its use was probably suggested by the earlier practice of miners in the area who regularly ingested lithomarge as well as a fine clay from sandstone mines known as "stone butter." *Kieselgur,* a chalky clay containing a great deal of calcium, was also eaten during various sieges of the fortress of Wittenberg during the eighteenth century. The eating of edible clays during famines has been recorded as well in Sweden, Finland, France, and Italy — in some instances as recently as the nineteenth century.

Many American Indians also ingested clays as survival "food" during famines and, according to numerous records, the Chinese ate particular types of earth identified as "stone meal" to keep from starving. Again, these were usually white clays, possibly identical with the *Kieselgur* of Germany and high in calcium. The clays were often powdered and mixed with rice or wheat before being baked or steamed. In some places, clays have been used as a portable, emergency food supply. On long journeys the natives of Borneo, for example, carry both red ocher and white oleaginous (oily) clays, which they claim are extremely nourishing. In parts of Africa, the Middle East, New Guinea, and Australia where clays have been eaten as a regular food, the habit is universally believed to have originated in times of severe famine.

People have eaten other, rather unique sorts of earth besides clay to appease hunger. Notably, the Mandja of Congo and Zaire collect earth from termites' nests during times of famine and mix it with water and powdered tree bark. The earth is said to literally "melt in the mouth" and is sometimes referred to as "delikatessen" earth. Both termite and ant earths have been found to be unusually high in many essential minerals, a fact which may very well explain why Moroccan women will sometimes ingest earth from an ant's nest to improve lactation.

Child-bearing women are perhaps the most frequent eaters of clays and dirts, invariably choosing earths that are rich in the mineral nutrition necessary to pregnancy and lactation. Various clays eaten by pregnant women in Africa contain significant amounts of calcium, copper, iron, magnesium, manganese, and zinc, depending on their source. Throughout the world women especially ingest clays rich in calcium and iron. Just as lactating rats increase their calcium consumption in experimental situations, and calcium-deficient mammals in the wild eat bones, it is likely that child-bearing women also "instinctively" select foods that are high in calcium — including calcium-rich clays. Direct evidence of food selection for sodium and iron has certainly been documented in human beings lacking these essential elements. This lends credence to the practice of pregnant women in Indonesia, who ingest the iron-rich *ampo* because, they say, "their fetus is fond of it."

Of course, any reasons given for such unusual diets must be taken, as geophagy expert Bernard Laufer once said, "with a grain of salt." Mineral deficiencies clearly do not drive all, or even a majority, of geophagical habits, no matter what people claim. A quite different but also very common use of edible clays has been to detoxify foods that would otherwise be inedible or poisonous. Acorns have been a staple food wherever oak trees are found, but untreated, they have such high concentrations of tannins (the same chemicals used to tan hides) that they are inedible as such by human beings. Most cultures have learned that boiling the acorns in several batches of water removes enough of the tannins to allow the nuts to be eaten. The Pomo Indians of California, however, developed a different detoxification technique. They mixed about one part clay with ten to twenty parts acorn meal, then baked the mixture as a bread. Poverty-stricken peasants in Sardinia made a similar acorn-clay bread up until a few decades ago. Recent studies have shown that heating the acorn meal in the presence of clay chemically neutralizes the tannins.

Detoxification also appears to have been the rationale for eating clay with other foods. Clays are included in many American Indian recipies that contain berries or tubers that would otherwise be noxious. The Hopi, Zuni, Pueblo, and Oraibi Indians of America's Southwest, for example, used to eat a small amount of white clay with the wild potato *Solanum fendleri,* which contains enough alkaloids to be poisonous when eaten raw or unskinned. Chemical studies of these "potato clays" has shown that they adsorb, or chemically bind with, very large amounts of the alkaloids, and thus prevent them from escaping from the gut into the bloodstream. The Aymara and Quechua people of the Andes Mountains of Bolivia and Peru continue to prepare wild potatoes with clay to this day. They say that the clay cuts the bitterness of the potatoes; their tongue tells them that the alkaloids have been neutralized. More fascinating still, Timothy Johns has argued that since all wild potatoes are poisonous to humans, the domestication of the modern potato from its native roots may actually have *required* geophagy at first.

Clays have also been important as medicines; the premodern Chinese may hold the record for the number of distinct uses. The sixteenth-century Chinese physician Li Shih-chen, for example, listed sixty-one pharmacological uses for clays, muds, and other earths in his *Pen-ts'ao kang-mu,* treating conditions from malnutrition to infection to diarrhea. Most other cultures have had more limited medical uses for earths. The ancient Greeks used soil dug from the island of Samos to treat people who were vomiting blood. The tenth-century Persian physician Rhazes prescribed the white clay of Nishapur for nausea and vomiting, and for centuries the Sudanese have ingested a clay called *tureba,* which is rich in sodium bicarbonate, for indigestion. Some American Indian tribes similarly cured bellyaches with small amounts of clay.

Clays are still being used as medicines today. The Toba-Batak of Sumatra claim that eating clay stops the vomiting associated with morning sickness in pregnant women. Many Nigerian tribes prescribe local clays for morning sickness, intestinal parasites, diarrhea, and dysentery, as do peoples throughout Asia and Australia. And in Indonesia *ampo* is used to cure nutritional disorders such as chlorosis, a form of anemia, and pica, the craving and eating of unnatural substances in general. From a Westerner's perspective, this last remedy is like treating an overindulgence in beer by substituting wine, since eating clay instead of mortar or charcoal, as occurs in pica, hardly seems an improvement. Yet because *ampo* is culturally accepted by the Indonesians, while other forms of pica are not, it is deemed expedient.

Both the Chinese and the Europeans also used medicinal clays to counteract the effects of poison. Terra sigillata, for example, was used to treat stomachaches due to illness as well as to ill will. Modern analyses of the clay banks from which terra sigillata and other "sealed earths" were produced show that they would in fact have been effective against many poisons, including those produced by bacteria in the gut. Clays have the ability to bind up materials that are ionized, or electrically charged, as many poisons are, especially those containing metals such as mercury or lead. In binding the poison, the clay releases an equal number of ions in a process called cation exchange. The cation-exchange capacity becomes a measure of how much of a particular poison the clay can adsorb. Modern analysis has shown that the amount of terra sigillata ingested by the prisoner at Baden in 1581 was almost exactly the amount necessary to neutralize the mercuric chloride he had eaten minutes before. There is, therefore, every reason to believe that his treatment really was successful and that terra sigillata was a useful antidote to many poisons. Forty years ago at least one pharmacologist even suggested that clays or synthetic versions called cation-exchange resins be used in preference to charcoal and milk as household antidotes for heavy-metal poisons.

The difficulty with assessing geophagy is that, like so many other folk medicines, it is like the Scottish claymore, a two-edged sword: for every outstanding benefit there is also a very deadly danger. In the American South ingested clays have generally been found to have such high levels of salt and low levels of potassium that they actually contribute to high blood pressure and a condition called hypokalemia, or potassium deficiency. In large amounts some clays cause vomiting and diarrhea, whether used medically for those purposes, as among the Mekeo of Oceania, or otherwise. The Mekeo also use certain clays instead of salt, thus depriving themselves of a much-needed nutrient in their diet. Moreover, clays low in nutritive value may actually bind up necessary ions such as calcium, zinc, and iron by the same process of cation exchange that makes them so useful as antidotes to poisons. Some ingested clays *may*, in short, cause malnutrition.

There is absolutely no doubt that a very good correlation exists between mineral deficiencies and geophagy, but whether the ingestion of earth is a corrective measure or a cause of malnutrition has not been decided by the experts. Perhaps the issue cannot be decided, since some earths contribute to nutrition and others detract from it. An additional problem is that eating earth not only takes away hunger pangs, it can also take away the desire for appropriate food. Ingesting too much clay or dirt can lead to anemia, stunted growth, and even outright starvation regardless of the nutrients in the soil. To make matters worse, geophagy appears to be addictive. Many people who take up clay eating find it nearly impossible to stop. While a bite or two a day may do little harm, more can create enteroliths, literally "stones that block the intestines," and eventually cause death.

In some areas of the world, eating earth also increases the risk of disease from infestation and infection; parasitic worms and the bacteria that cause typhoid and other waterborne diseases can live in edible muds and clays. Even eating earths to ameliorate an illness can carry the risk of worsening it. For instance, using clays to help stop diarrhea, while symptomatically useful, can actually complicate or obscure the disease process. The most dangerous aspect of diarrhea is not the runny stool per se, but water and salt loss. If water and electrolyte balance are not restored in diarrhetic patients, simply firming up their stool will not save them.

The risks are very real and have played at least one very sad role in history. Many slaves captured in Africa and shipped to South, Central, and North America brought along their habit of eating various earths for nutritional and medicinal purposes. In many cases they were not able to locate appropriate clays for their needs but continued to ingest earth anyway. Slave owners were almost universally appalled by the habit, not only because it offended their sensibilities but because it hurt their pocketbooks. They quickly noted that earth-eating slaves were malnourished, weak, dull, and generally unhealthy. Indeed, it was believed that they ate dirt as a way of committing suicide. Many of them certainly died from their habit. In consequence, slave owners tried every means possible to stamp out geophagy, including whippings, torture, mouth-locks, and even special cone-shaped masks that prevented eating at any but observed and controlled times. None of these methods worked. Geophagy is still practiced today by a much larger proportion of African Americans than of any other ethnic group, and the habit is thought to contribute to their much higher incidence of malnutrition. Cultural habits have long-term health consequences that cannot easily be reversed.

The misuses, abuses, and dangers of geophagy cannot be overlooked, but there is nonetheless a subterranean vein of validity in the practice. We still use clays for detoxification in very much the same way that the preparers of terra sigillata intended. In fact, there is a type of clay called fuller's earth that is still prescribed today to treat people who have ingested a poison for which no specific antidote is known, such as the herbicides paraquat and diquat. Fuller's earth gets its name from the ancient process of "fulling" wool to clean it of dirt and oil. It consists essentially of aluminum silicates and is used in industry, in much the same way as charcoal, to filter and decontaminate. It has occasionally even been used medicinally to help adsorb the endotoxins, or bacterial poisons, produced by severe infections such as inflammatory bowel syndrome. Fuller's earth is also recommended as a medical antidote for chemical and biological warfare agents.

Significantly, all of the clays traditionally used by American Indian and African tribes for treating gastrointestinal distress that have so far been analyzed have been predominately kaolin-type clays, like fuller's earth. Analyses of the particular clays used by American Indians for acorn meal preparation have shown that they rival fuller's earth in their ability to adsorb tannins. This property would also have justified the use of these clays in the past as antidiarrhetics, provided, of course, that care was taken to prevent dehydration.

We don't want to make too many claims for clays. Despite a number of valid indications, the medicinal use of earth is manifestly unusual today. The real question is whether *you* have ever ingested some earthy substance, and the answer is almost surely yes. It may be somewhat of a stretch to suggest that eating nutritious earths is the origin of mineral supplements, for there are many other sources of essential minerals in our diets, such as vegetables and meats. Yet we add reduced iron, zinc oxide, calcium phosphate, cupric oxide, magnesium oxide, and potassium iodide to our complete multivitamin pills and to our cereals in much the same way that people used to add a bite of mineral-rich clay to their diet. Granted, we now make most of these mineral additives industrially instead of having to find them at a salt lick or clay bank. But if we pop a pill instead of eating a few grams of termite-mound earth, the difference is one of detail rather than of kind.

There is no stretch at all, however, in suggesting that you have ingested earth if you have ever taken a common antacid or buffered pain reliever or an antidiarrheal such as Kaopectate. Many antacids can trace their histories back to the use of magnesia, or magnesium oxide, which occurs in nature as the mineral periclase and is named after the "stones of Magnesia" in Greece, where it was originally found. Hundreds of years ago Macedonians added magnesia to their bread, considering it a cheap form of nutrition. The mineral magnesium is, in fact, necessary to good health, and at least two pharmaceutical companies prepare and sell magnesium oxide supplements for the treatment of magnesium deficiencies associated with the use of diuretics, digitalis, and various chemotherapies. It is worth noting, however, that in the general population magnesium deficiency is extremely rare. Today magnesium oxide and its close cousin magnesium hydroxide, both common constituents of the clays our ancestors ate for stomach upsets, are used most frequently to treat indigestion. These can be found in such common over-the-counter medications as Maalox, Mylanta, Di-Gel, and, of course, Phillips' milk of magnesia. Moreover, the buffering agents in Bufferin, buffered Excedrin, and Cama Arthritis Pain Reliever include both magnesium oxide and magnesium carbonate as well as calcium carbonate.

Calcium carbonate is another widely used antacid, found in products such as Di-Gel, Rolaids, and Tums. It is also prescribed as a calcium supplement to help build strong bones and teeth or to reverse osteoporosis and is the main ingredient in Caltrate, Os-Cal tablets, and various other calcium preparations. Its naturally occurring form is chalk, most often formed from fossilized seashells, and as such is to be found in *Kieselgur* and many other edible rocks from around the world. Chalk won't make a meal complete, but starving people may indeed have benefited from its ingestion in the past, just as people who are lactose intolerant or suffering from bone loss today can benefit from calcium supplements. And, of course, calcium carbonate is a tried and true remedy for stomachaches. Chalk up another success for geopharmacy!

Kaopectate is another common medicine derived from the earth. It is essentially a combination of two folk remedies for gastrointestinal distress: pectin, found in high amounts in fruits such as cooked blackberries, which some American Indians ate to treat diarrhea, and kaolin, a white clay made up primarily of hydrated aluminum silicate. Kaolin, sometimes called china or porcelain clay, is used in making fine porcelain, bricks, Portland cement, plaster, and many other materials. Its gut-calming effects no doubt explain why some potters have reported nibbling on their clay while they work, not only in the West but in all pottery-making cultures. Kaolin is also found in such prescription medications for diarrhea as Kaolin-Pectin Suspension, Donnagel-PG, and Parepectolin Suspension. Interestingly, kaolin is still prepared for medicinal purposes just as it has been for millennia: it is washed with water and sieved to remove sand and other particles, then allowed to precipitate into its pure and ingestible form. Today we stamp the package with the manufacturer's seal instead of stamping lozenges of dried clay, and we sometimes camouflage the earth with colorful dyes, but in essence it's still geophagy, pure and simple.

So if you ever wondered why some antacids and antidiarrheal medicines taste (or perhaps *feel* is a better word) a bit earthy, the secret's out. Modern medicine has muddied the waters surrounding the origins of these treatments so well that most of us don't even realize we have eaten good china as well as eaten off it.

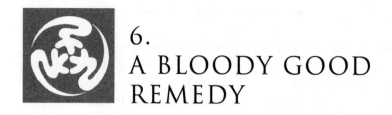

6.
A BLOODY GOOD
REMEDY

*Experience must, indeed, as Hippocrates says in
his first aphorism, be fallacious if we decide that a
means of treatment, sanctioned by the use of between
two and three thousand years, and upheld by the
authority of the ablest men of past times, is finally
and forever given up . . . He would be a very bold
man who, after looking carefully through the history
of the past, would venture to assert that bleeding
will not be profitably employed any more.*
— W. Mitchell Clarke, M.D., 1875

MENTION DRAWING BLOOD for testing
purposes and most people cringe. Mention drawing blood as a form of medical therapy and most people
shudder in disbelief. But it has not always been so. Consider this.
Sometime in the early 1800s a ship's surgeon named Lionel Wafer
observed some Central American Indians shoot little arrows into
a patient's back, piercing the skin and drawing blood in small
spurts. Far from being dismayed, Wafer understood perfectly what
they were doing. And at the first opportunity he demonstrated in
turn the favored technique of bloodletting in his own native England. When a sick Indian woman came to him for care, "I bound
up her arm with a piece of bark," wrote Wafer, "and with my lancet
breathed a vein . . . and I drew off about 12 ounces and bound up
her arm, and desired she might rest till the next day; by which
means the fever abated and she had not another fit."

The woman's recovery gained Wafer a certain renown among the Indians, but what are we to make of his bloodletting — or theirs? The idea of "breathing," or opening, a vein and drawing blood to make a sick person well seems preposterous and cruel. Yet bloodletting as a cure has one of the oldest pedigrees in medical history. More than two thousand years before Wafer pulled out his lancet, a specialized bloodletting tool, a Hindu doctor on the Indian subcontinent chanted prayers as he prepared to slit the temporal vein of his patient "to the depth of a barley corn." The man suffered from an unattended leg wound, which had turned putrid and was full of maggots. The doctor had removed the "worms due to flies" and cleaned the wound, but now, two days later, the man had returned with fever, a swollen foot, and a throbbing headache. To the doctor, the indications for bleeding were unmistakable. Following his directions, the patient took up the required position, pressing closed fists to either side of his neck and holding his breath. The doctor cut, and blood flowed.

Did the treatment have anything to do with the complaint? Bloodletting, whether practiced by "primitive" or "civilized" peoples, strikes many of us today as perhaps the most useless, misguided, and barbaric of past medical practices. Except that the barbarians are also us. Just a few decades ago, Drs. George Burch and Nicolas DePasquale, attending physicians at the Charity Hospital of Louisiana, performed yet another bloodletting. They examined a sixty-nine-year-old doctor who was exhibiting symptoms of angina pectoris, severe but short-lived attacks of chest pain. Burch and DePasquale prescribed coronary dilators, drugs that increase blood flow to the heart. The patient continued to complain of "heaviness in his chest" and the feeling that another attack would occur at any moment. Burch and DePasquale then bled the man and the "heaviness" disappeared. They bled him again, several times, and the patient's long-standing high blood pressure returned to normal.

The old doctor was so impressed with the results of the bleeding that whenever he felt the preliminary symptoms of angina he voluntarily returned and requested venesection — another word for the drawing of blood by opening a vein. Burch and DePasquale obliged. Nor was he the only one to ask for this treatment. These doctors bled many patients with heart disease, including a woman in whom a persistent angina pectoris had ceased after a serious episode of internal hemorrhage. It was her heartfelt opinion that "bleeding was good for her" and would be good for others suffering the same attacks of chest pain. Burch and DePasquale obviously concurred.

Was the bloodletting really responsible for the cure in these or any other cases down the ages? It seems more plausible to argue that relief for Burch and DePasquale's patients was, instead, spontaneous and unrelated to treatment; that the Indian woman recovered in spite of losing a cup and a half of blood just when she needed it most; that the Hindu's infected leg wound could not possibly have been favorably affected by bloodletting in the head. Bleeding for fever, inflammation, or pain in the chest just doesn't seem rational or right. "Medicine," one physician and scholar recently wrote, "never produced a greater absurdity." Seen from this point of view, bloodletting was indeed a venal practice.

If bloodletting is considered nothing more than corrupt chicanery, however, then nearly all physicians in the past were charlatans. The truth is that for most of recorded history bloodletting was, as one European practitioner put it in 1830, "not only the most powerful and important, but the most generally used, of all our remedies." At one time or another nearly all societies and cultures have removed blood from the body for therapeutic purposes. Evidence of its use can be found in the ancient Hebrew, Greek, Arabic, Hindu, and Babylonian civilizations. Thorns, fish teeth, and sharpened stones found at archaeological sites support the speculation that bloodletting is in fact prehistoric and dates back at least as far as the Stone Age.

The practice persisted for thousands of years, especially where traditional cultures resisted change. Within the past two hundred years missionaries and ethnologists have reported bloodletting in isolated areas all over the world, from the Polynesian Islands to remote parts of Africa. On the Pacific island of Ponape,

for example, painful bruises were tapped with a shark or barra-
cuda tooth to let the "bad blood" flow out. The cure for a rapid
heartbeat in Zimbabwe involved placing a locust on numerous
shallow cuts to the chest and allowing it to drink the blood and fly
away. And not many years ago in Belize "an old Mayan bush doctor" healed chronic migraine by puncturing a man's forehead in
three places with a stingray spine. As the dark, frothy blood fell to
the floor, the pain disappeared. "There you see your sickness on
the floor," explained the bush doctor. "I've taken out the congested old blood blocked in your head, causing headaches. Blood
should run like a river — clear, clean and free."

We infer the ancestry of the bush doctor's remedy from the
ancestry of the tool — stingray spines have been found in ancient
Mayan tombs. But his explanation was also archaic. The Mayan
healer's words sounded very much like those of an ancient Egyptian or Greek physician. The Egyptians also removed "bad blood"
by scarifying, or making shallow cuts in the skin. Eventually a more
elaborate theory became associated with the Greek physician Hippocrates, who taught that all disease was caused by an imbalance
in the body's four humors: blood, phlegm, yellow bile, and black
bile. One way to restore balance was to let blood. Galen, a Greek
physician who lived in the second century A.D., performed venesection for practically every disease, especially feverish ones.

Because Galen's texts had a profound effect on European
medicine, bloodletting became standard medical therapy for the
next 1500 years — in fact, a cure-all. People were bled for all
serious illnesses and for any number of lesser complaints. In addition to fever, these included cough, fatigue, insomnia, apoplexy,
angina pectoris, asthma, vomiting blood, bruises, coughs, tuberculosis, contusions, diseases of the hip and knee joints, deafness,
delirium and lunacy, dropsy, epilepsy, dizziness, gout, headaches,
inflammations of the eyes and lungs, drunkenness, lumbago, measles, numbness of the limbs, pleurisy, palsy, rheumatism, sciatica,
shortness of breath, and sore throat.

Bloodletting was at times so commonplace and copious that
historians have referred to the "vampirism" of certain medical cir-

cles. One Italian practitioner boasted that he had bled a woman 1309 times in the last four years of her life, almost once a day! How much blood the good doctor drew each time is unknown. Galen had advised removing as little as seven ounces or as much as a pound and a half (around a pint and a half, or 750 milliliters). Usually smaller amounts were drawn several times over a number of days. By the eighteenth and nineteenth centuries the volume tended to be greater. One massive bleeding (900 milliliters) might drain nearly a quart, around one fifth of the body's total blood volume. As much as a fourth or a third of a person's blood supply may have been drawn as physicians attempted to "bleed to syncope," or collapse. They knowingly trod a fine line here; if more blood were taken, shock would ensue, leading to death. (For contrast, consider that current American Red Cross practice is to allow a person to be bled of one pint every three months.)

One might objectively expect that if bloodletting had no therapeutic value whatsoever, it would not have been practiced in so many cultures and would not have lasted so long in our own. But what was its true value? Two avenues of present-day medical practice and research, one clinical, the other experimental, have revealed some answers. Not only is bloodletting still being used today in the treatment of certain diseases, its physiological effects on the body have been explored in depth — and with surprisingly positive results.

One of the most important clues concerning the possible beneficial effects of bloodletting has come from the work of Canadian physiologist Norman Kasting. Through the 1980s Kasting was involved in medical research on the control of fever by regulatory centers in the brain. In particular, he found that the hormone vasopressin, when injected into the brains of experimental animals, reversed or prevented the rise of body temperature typical of fever. Kasting knew that the natural release of vasopressin was stimulated by dehydration and hemorrhage. The next logical step was to determine whether therapeutic bloodletting would cause sufficient release of vasopressin to have an antipyretic or fever-reducing effect. Experiments with feverish sheep and rats proved this effect, but was it true for humans? For ethical reasons such an experiment could not be done, so Kasting turned to the past for experimental insight.

Dipping into the medical literature from the early Greeks to the late-nineteenth-century Europeans, Kasting found, to his surprise, a common thread: physicians in the past often drew blood explicitly to reduce fever. In case after case across the centuries, doctors reported that immediately following a copious loss of blood, patients experienced relief from the heat and pain of fever. Galen drew blood and "slaughtered the fever." In the eighteenth century the physician Hugh Smith let blood and "diminished . . . the heat of the body . . . immediately injurious to life." Bloodletting proved especially efficacious in treating the tropical fevers encountered by Europeans in Africa and the Americas. And by the end of the 1800s C. A. Wunderlich, who produced the first great study of variations in human temperature using the newly invented clinical thermometer, reported that "the immediate result of a considerable loss of blood is almost always a considerable reduction of temperature."

Kasting concluded from the historical evidence that bloodletting was indeed an effective antipyretic stimulus in human beings. But did the reduction of fever actually "cure" disease? We know that a mild fever can be beneficial. We also know that a fever that spikes too high poses grave danger to the brain and other tissues. Kasting speculated that bloodletting may directly benefit the sick and contribute to their healing in three ways. First, the loss of blood stimulates a reduction of fever, which protects sensitive body tissues from harm and relieves discomfort, allowing rest and sleep. Second, loss of blood also lowers the level of iron in the body. Because many bacteria need iron in order to thrive and reproduce in the body, reducing this nutrient may aid in recovery. And, lastly, loss of blood causes the pituitary gland to release several hormones (one of which is vasopressin) that stimulate immune function.

We are left with the exciting proposition that bloodletting not only reduced potentially dangerous fever but also inhibited bacteria and boosted the immune system. The Hindu doctor and ship surgeon Wafer may indeed have "cured" their feverish patients, not only of fever but of the underlying disease. The stronger link between bloodletting and fever reduction, however, helps explain the general demise of this treatment just as simpler, less risky means of controlling fever became widely available. The discovery of sodium salicylate (extracted from willow leaves) in 1876 and the manufacture of acetylsalicylic acid (aspirin) in 1899 coincide roughly with the end of bloodletting for severe fevers such as scarlet fever, typhus, yellow fever, measles, and meningitis. Why bleed when it was easier to take a powder or pop a pill?

At the same time the growth of skeptical inquiry caused doctors to discontinue the drawing of blood in diseases unrelated to fever. By the 1890s medical distrust of phlebotomy had become so marked that some of its valid uses were in danger of being lost. "During the first five decades of this century, the profession bled too much," observed William Osler, preeminent physician of the late nineteenth century, "but during the last decades we have certainly bled too little." Osler knew from experience and conscientious study that certain diseases, such as aneurysm and heart failure, had at that time no other or better treatment than venesection. He refused to delete the therapy from his textbooks, which were still being reprinted in the early 1900s. For this reason he was partially responsible for the "rediscovery" of phlebotomy in the treatment of these diseases about fifty years ago.

Aortic aneurysm is a serious condition in which a pulsating blood-filled sac bulges from the abnormally weakened wall of the aorta, the major artery that leaves the heart. Marked by pain, faintness, shortness of breath, and swelling of the neck, face, and arms, such an aneurysm can rupture at any time, causing massive internal hemorrhage. Physicians in the seventeenth and eighteenth centuries tried to reduce the sac with zealous bleedings and a near-starvation diet. Unfortunately, most people put off such drastic treatment until their suffering was great and death imminent. Since aortic aneurysm was then a common consequence of syphilis, the cure must have seemed a fitting recompense for the sin. And since many patients died while undergoing treatment, venesection for aneurysm disappeared along with the general demise of bloodletting in the latter half of the nineteenth century.

However, in the late 1930s the old "cure" was unearthed once more. Dr. Eugene Marzullo, an attending physician at Long Island College Hospital in New York, performed emergency venesection on an Italian immigrant with a large aneurysm near bursting that bulged several inches from the upper chest. "Immediate and striking relief resulted," Marzullo later reported, "and I was encouraged to repeat it in an effort to establish a cure. . . . [V]enesection, 500 cc at a time, was done over a period of two months." In the 1950s some American doctors, citing Marzullo, who had cited Osler, once again took up vigorous phlebotomy to relieve the severe pulsing pain of aneurysm and in some cases to reduce the sac itself. Sometimes the relief was only temporary. But under the best of circumstances the treatment promoted the coagulation of blood in the sac, thereby closing it off and rendering it harmless. This resurgence of phlebotomy for aneurysm was, however, very brief. The use of penicillin to treat syphilis drastically reduced the number of aneurysms caused by that disease, while new methods of surgically correcting aneurysm made bloodletting obsolete.

A similar resurgence of phlebotomy in the treatment of congestive heart failure was also quelled by subsequent medical advances. Congestive heart failure is a condition characterized by shortness of breath, swelling at the ankles, palpitations, and coughing up of watery sputum. During the 1950s researchers determined that in many cases an increase in blood volume contributed to the inadequate pumping action of the diseased heart. The inefficient blood circulation led, in turn, to congestion of the lungs and liver and distention of the veins of the neck. By lowering the volume of blood, phlebotomy relieved the ailing heart and restored circulation to the congested tissues, thus reducing the risk of life-threatening pulmonary edema (fluid in the lungs). In the 1960s the introduction of effective diuretics offered physicians an alternative means of decreasing blood volume, and thus edema, and bloodletting was once again set aside; it is now used only when diuretics do not work or are contraindicated.

Phlebotomy for angina pectoris is a story with the same plot. Although no one knew exactly why, the loss of as little as three or four ounces of blood brought prompt relief to angina patients. With this knowledge we can see that Drs. Burch and DePasquale were following a time-honored treatment in the 1960s. Nor was the use of blood-sipping locusts in Zimbabwe to treat chest pains far-fetched — though the therapeutic agent was surely the bleeding, not the bugs. But as in so many other cases, drugs made bloodletting for angina less attractive to patients and physicians alike. The amyl nitrites, introduced in 1867, took the place of phlebotomy precisely because they seemed to mimic its pain-killing result. In 1970 American researchers investigating more closely the effect of nitrites on heart and pulse also studied venesection and found that it not only reduced blood volume, it actually decreased pressure in the resting heart and lowered its need for oxygen. Since angina results from a deficient supply of oxygen to the heart, bleeding was sufficient to relieve or prevent attacks of pain. Amyl nitrites performed a similar function by increasing peripheral blood flow (causing, among other things, a flushed skin) and lowering internal blood volume.

The resurgence of phlebotomy in the 1950s and '60s proved, if nothing else, that thousands of years of practice had not been totally in vain. So compelling was this realization at the time that the medical profession wondered, as one editorial in the *Journal of the American Medical Association* in 1963 put it, whether or not "an ancient procedure [was] turning modern." A trickle of recognized uses had become a stream. By the early 1960s researchers were exploring the role of erythrocytosis — an abnormal increase in the number of red blood cells — in angina pectoris and in heart attack. In patients suffering from these diseases, bloodletting alleviated chest pain not only by reducing volume pressure on the heart but by reducing the overabundance of red blood cells. This, in turn, appeared to reduce clotting or "sludging" of the blood and to promote circulation to the heart itself. Thus, according to the same editorial, the old notion of "plethora" as a deleterious abundance of blood, when understood scientifically, was also a meaningful modern concept that could be effectively addressed by bloodletting.

Today phlebotomy is not usually considered as a treatment for angina pectoris, heart attack, or congestive heart failure because we have effective drugs and surgical interventions to deal with these problems, but it does remain the primary treatment for certain disorders that can lead to heart problems. These include polycythemia vera, hemochromatosis, and porphyria cutanea tarda. Polycythemia vera, primarily a disease of old age, is characterized in part by an uncontrolled erythrocytosis. The letting of 400 to 500 milliliters of blood two to four times a year or, in severe cases, weekly, serves to reduce the plethora of blood cells, thereby reducing the risk of spontaneous bleeding or, conversely, of blood clotting. Symptoms such as headache, dizziness, blurred vision, ringing in the ears, palpitations, and memory loss are greatly relieved by this therapy. Circulation improves, and stress on the heart decreases. When started early enough, phlebotomy can prevent a complicating leukemia and extend life expectancy ten or twelve years.

Porphyria cutanea tarda is an enzyme deficiency disease that affects the production of hemoglobin, resulting in the excessive accumulation of intermediate proteins known as porphyrins. Unlike the more infamous inherited forms of porphyria, such as the acute intermittent form that caused the madness of King George III of England, porphyria cutanea tarda is generally considered an acquired disease brought on by excessive alcohol abuse, birth control medications, or other toxic exposures that interfere with porphyrin metabolism. The disease presents with skin photosensitivity, skin lesions, darkening of the skin, and hirsutism (abnormal hair growth), and most patients suffer damage to the liver caused by high levels of iron. Indeed, it has been suggested that alcohol abuse coupled with an iron-rich diet — both common among peoples as disparate as Bantus and Italians — predisposes to the de-

velopment of porphyria cutanea tarda. The removal of 500 milliliters of blood every two to four weeks eventually depletes the
overload of iron, and the symptoms of disease go into remission.
Avoidance of alcohol or other chemical triggers and additional
phlebotomies as needed can prevent premature death from liver
failure.

Phlebotomy is also a primary treatment for hemochromatosis, an inherited abnormality that causes the gut to absorb too
much iron. By the age of fifty or sixty a person with hemochromatosis has accumulated twenty or thirty times the normal amount of
iron in the liver, the heart, the pancreas, and other organs, all of
which show signs of serious degeneration. Complaints of weakness, lassitude, and vague abdominal pain are typical early signs
that are easily overlooked; the disease often progresses to a "classic
triad" of liver disease, diabetes, and heart failure. An aggressive
course of phlebotomy can reduce the overload of iron, halt or
reverse organ degeneration, and extend life expectancy twenty
years. Doctors remove 400 to 500 milliliters of blood per week for
two or three years until the patient's iron stores are depleted and
mild anemia sets in. Thereafter they treat the disease with four to
six phlebotomies per year for the patient's entire lifetime. Talk
about medical vampires! In hemochromatosis, if not polycythemia
vera and porphyria cutanea tarda, modern physicians rival the
bloodletting rates of yesteryear!

Given what we now know about valid medical uses of phlebotomy in this century, we can understand that it was a rational
therapy supported by empirical results in the past. To begin with,
the heart and blood diseases that respond to bloodletting have
always been quite common. Angina pectoris affects about 3.5 percent of the population of Great Britain. Congestive heart failure
affects about 1 percent of Americans. Less than .5 percent of
the U.S. population currently suffers from aortic aneurysm. Estimates for hemochromatosis in the populations of Western countries range from less than one in four hundred to about one in a
hundred persons. Anglo-Saxons as a group may have rates as high
as three in a hundred. Porphyria cutanea tarda occurs in the

absence of environmental triggers in less than .2 percent of European populations, but in populations exposed to iron-rich alcohols or certain toxic chemicals, its incidence can rise as high as 2 percent. Polycythemia vera occurs in about .02 percent of European peoples and is thus negligible.

Given these figures we might expect 6 percent of today's population in the West to be suffering from one or another of these diseases at any one time, and our forebears probably had these illnesses in similar proportions. Some complaints may actually have been more prevalent. We speculate that cooking in iron pots and pans may have caused the iron overload associated with hemochromatosis and porphyria cutanea tarda to be much more common. Chronic alcoholism, especially rampant in eighteenth-century Europe and America, may also have helped boost the rates of porphyria cutanea tarda. Aortic aneurysm was highly associated with syphilis, a disease endemic in the preantibiotic age. Heart disease in general has declined in recent years as a result of modern preventive medicine, leading us to expect higher rates in the past; however, congestive heart failure and angina pectoris may actually have been less common then, at least among the poorer classes of European society. Both are rare in populations suffering from malnutrition, parasitic infection, and chronic anemia.

In addition to people with diseases known to respond to bloodletting, we must add those who were treated for fevers — perhaps the most common premodern use of phlebotomy. We will guess that illnesses characterized by fevers affected several percent of a population at any one time. Altogether, this means that if a doctor bled a hundred people at random in the mid-eighteenth or early nineteenth century, we might expect between six and ten of them to have been suffering from some disease that responds observably well to the phlebotomy! Of course, those people who actually sought medical care were not a random group: they were sick. Many had symptoms such as fever, chest pain, lassitude, or dropsy, all of which were indications for bloodletting, so our 6 to 10 percent figure is unrealistically low. The real figure for that

proportion of a doctor's patients who would have responded em-
pirically to venesection must have been at least several times more,
say anywhere from 20 to 40 percent.

This puts phlebotomy in a new light. Any medical procedure
that benefits even 20 percent of patients treated is powerful stuff.
Today we routinely ingest drugs and undergo surgery on the basis
of similar odds. Only thirty-eight out of a hundred people suffering a ruptured aneurysm, for example, will make it to the hospital
alive, and of those, only about twenty will survive emergency surgery. Yet we would never suggest that because only twenty percent
survive the medical intervention of ambulance service and surgical repair we ought not to bother with the attempt. Bloodletting
probably worked at least as often to eliminate fever, pain, or dropsical swelling. This is not to say that every use or even most uses of
bloodletting in the past were scientifically sound, but enough patients through the ages probably did experience sufficient immediate or even long-term relief due to the controlled loss of blood
to convince even skeptical doctors to continue the practice.

One final use of phlebotomy remains tantalizingly on the
fence between nonsense and good sense. For centuries many
Europeans practiced prophylactic bleeding to maintain their
health and extend life. Monks bled themselves several times a year
to prevent disease, as did many others in the medieval period. The
custom continued through the fifteenth and sixteenth centuries,
when advice on bloodletting as part of a healthy lifestyle circulated
in learned books and common almanacs alike. Thereafter the
prophylactic use of phlebotomy waxed and waned, until it reached
new heights in the early nineteenth century. The English in particular practiced biannual bloodlettings in such numbers that at
times the hospitals were overwhelmed. Persons "bled to faintness"
were said to fill the halls and wards. Later in the century the
American physician Henry Bowditch acknowledged that patients
often asked him to "breathe a vein" as part of an annual ritual of
health maintenance; he claimed that he refused. In any case, as
pills and dietary regimens made headway in the American health
market, the custom slowly went the way of therapeutic venesec-

tion. In the early 1900s only European immigrants continued to seek the prophylactic bleedings that modern medical culture had deemed nonsensical.

Studies of women's risks of heart disease and iron deficiency, combined with the twentieth-century inventions of blood donation and blood banking, may change this view of preventive venesection. While no one these days would recommend a return to bloodletting as a general remedy, several researchers have suggested that regular phlebotomy may actually be beneficial to one's health. According to Jerome Sullivan and R. B. Lauffer, one of the major puzzles of modern living is the observed sex difference in rates of heart disease: premenopausal women are far less likely than men to suffer and die of heart attacks. There is no scientifically verified explanation for this phenomenon, though much investigation has been directed toward the role of female hormones.

Sullivan proposes alternatively that the female protective factor may very well be the monthly loss of menstrual blood, which naturally decreases the amount of iron in a woman's body. Indeed, women are much more likely than men to have iron-deficiency anemia. Once menopause begins, however, the level of iron in a woman's body rises, along with the risk of heart disease. Citing hemochromatosis as a model, Sullivan proposes that increasing levels of iron even modestly above the depleted or anemic state may predispose a person to heart disease. This theory would explain the higher risk of heart disease observed in men, postmenopausal women, and those who eat a great deal of red meat, which is rich in iron as well as cholesterol. According to Lauffer, it would also explain the benefits of exercise as a heart disease preventive, since regular aerobic exercise also lowers iron stores.

At present this connection between iron level and heart disease is largely theoretical, and existing data are contradictory. Letting blood affects not only the level of iron, after all, but also hormone and cholesterol levels and immune function. Other physiological systems may be affected as well, since recent studies have indicated that regular phlebotomy reduces blood pressure in

85

people suffering from resistant hypertension. The iron theory may be too simplistic, but it does raise an intriguing and easily tested possibility. Perhaps regular blood donations prolong the donor's life by decreasing the risk for heart attack or stimulating blood and immune functions. A small study undertaken in Italy in 1983 did find that the chances of living to age seventy-five were much higher for blood donors of both sexes than for those who had never donated blood. Of course, one study does not constitute a proof, but it is enough to make you think those medieval monks and nineteenth-century Britons were not faint-hearted fools after all.

Perhaps in the future the familiar Red Cross slogan "Help save lives" may be changed to something like "Help save lives and lengthen your own." That would not be too different from the old English adage "A bleeding in the spring is physic for a king." How ironic that we may be in a position to verify this claim long after bloodletting has been thoroughly discarded in all but a handful of disorders. Intriguing links between bloodletting and iron storage, bloodletting and immune function, bloodletting and longevity, beg for further investigation. At our most sanguine, we might even give credence to an old Mayan healer and look into the effect of cranial phlebotomy on migraine. If even a small bleeding can affect circulation to the heart in angina, why might it not affect circulation to the brain as well?

Despite its ancient and oft-discredited origins, phlebotomy is one of modern medicine's most important tools. When used by trained doctors for scientifically valid reasons, the risks are small and the benefits profound. Far from absurd, bloodletting is proving itself to be a bloody good remedy.

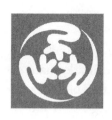

7.
HIRUDO THE HERO

I believe the secretions from bloodsucking animals
are to cardiovascular disease what penicillin was to
infectious disease.

— Roy Sawyer, Ph.D., 1991

FREAK ACCIDENTS can make for heroic medicine. One day in May of 1994 at a Los Angeles packaging company, a woman's long brown ponytail, usually tucked out of the way, suddenly swung forward into moving machinery. The blade of a huge industrial blender snagged the hair, ripping her scalp in one piece from her cranium. Almost at once paramedics arrived, bandaged the woman's bleeding head, and retrieved her scalp from the blender. Immediately they sealed it in a plastic bag and placed it in a container of ice, doubling the time — to twelve or maybe eighteen hours — that the amputated scalp would remain viable. Within three hours the woman arrived at the USC University Hospital, where surgeons were renowned for the replantation of amputated fingers and hands. They had never before reattached a scalp.

This lack of experience was hardly surprising, for the injury was rare and the procedure difficult. Indeed, it was not until the development of microsurgical techniques in the late 1970s that a scalp could be replanted with any hope of success. Peering through high-power microscopes, surgeons had learned to anastomose, or rejoin, blood vessels so small they were almost impossible to find. In this way they were able to reestablish the flow of freshly oxygenated arterial blood, without which the replanted tissue could not survive. However, if the veins remained inadequate or blocked, the replanted tissue swelled with stagnant, bluish, oxygen-depleted blood. Unreversed, this venous congestion led to tissue death. The challenge in microsurgery was to minimize and overcome venous congestion in the first five to ten postoperative days, until capillary return restored itself within the injured tissue. Between 1983 and May 1994, fewer than eighteen full scalp replantations had been successfully performed worldwide.

The intrepid surgeons at USC University Hospital picked up the gauntlet. Four hours after the accident, with only hours to go before the scalp died, the patient entered the operating room. While one surgical team prepared the scalp, cleaning it of hair and searching for blood vessels, another team unbandaged the patient's head and prepared the cranium for replantation. Then the grueling process of reattaching the scalp began. Most of the major blood vessels had been destroyed in the accident; the surgeons found only one artery and two veins. With meticulous care, they sewed them back together, using suture thinner than a human hair. After five hours of painstaking microanastomosis they reset a viable scalp in place.

The surgeons had completed their work well within the allotted time, but shortly after surgery, as feared and expected, an area of the scalp just above the patient's right ear showed signs of venous congestion. The surgeons had done all they could, which was a great deal. But draining the engorged tissue was a critical task fit for another sort of hero. The surgeons called on *Hirudo medicinalis,* a little guy flown in from New York just for this case.

Hirudo didn't look like a hero. He looked, well, like a worm. The nurse opened a jar and, brandishing a pair of tweezers, picked out a slippery, brownish-green leech about two inches long with a sucker at each end of its body. She touched the narrower mouth to a carefully marked spot on the dusky scalp. With its y-shaped jaw and hundreds of teeth, the leech bit painlessly through the patient's skin and promptly began to suck. In the next twenty to forty minutes it drew around 20 to 60 milliliters of blood — equal to nine times its body weight — out of the congested tissue. Swollen and satiated, the leech then dropped off and was removed, but the bite leaked an additional 15 to 30 milliliters of blood over several hours. For the next eight days new leeches were applied until finally capillary circulation reestablished itself throughout the wound. The scalp was saved.

It may be startling to see a lowly worm play such a mighty role in sophisticated medicine, but leeching is far from uncommon in replantation cases. The field of microsurgery is barely thirty years old, and for the last ten or fifteen years plastic and reconstructive surgeons have sucked up to bloodsuckers in a big way. Dozens and dozens of articles mention their use. Given this sudden interest, we might think that leeches were new to medicine. In fact, doctors have been stuck on these particular worms for as long as human beings have drawn blood for therapeutic purposes.

The cultural evidence is pictorial, textual, even lexical. A wall painting in an Egyptian tomb suggests that leeching to remove blood was an established practice in lands along the Nile more than 3000 years ago. The earliest known written record of bloodletting with leeches comes from India some 2000 years ago. The ancient Greeks applied leeches for headaches and numerous other ailments, and later the Romans used leeches to reduce black eyes and rectify imbalances among the humors of the body. The practice of leeching spread from these cradles of civilization into the farthest reaches of Europe, or developed independently. In medieval Britain healers used bloodsuckers so extensively that the word "leech," which derives from the Anglo-Saxon *loece,* "to heal," was applied to both doctor and worm, and "leechcraft" became synonymous with medicine.

By the seventeenth century the leech was as widely used in northern Europe as the lancet, and for all the same reasons. Any ailment managed by venesection was equally amenable (or so it was thought) to the leech. Then again, certain ailments, such as bruises, black eyes, headaches, insomnia, ulcers, obesity, and gout, were particularly treated with leeches because the tiny creatures drew blood directly from the affected tissues, often with visible local effects. Moreover, unlike venesection, which was confined to the location of favorable veins, leeching could be done virtually anywhere on the body. For example, the eighteenth-century British surgeon John Hunter applied leeches to the temples for inflammation of the eye, to the scrotum for testicles swollen by gonorrhea, and below the anus for inflammation of the bladder. Not only were these areas difficult if not impossible to lance, but, Hunter claimed, leeches accomplished the required bloodletting with less pain and irritation! Indeed, the leech was often preferred to the lancet for women and children who required a gentle withdrawal of blood.

The leech reached the peak of its popularity in Europe in the first half of the nineteenth century. Napoleon's military surgeon, François-Joseph Broussais, was one of the most prominent trendsetters. As a rule he advocated thirty to fifty leeches at a time, enough to draw one to one and a half quarts of blood, a massive bleeding! It was Broussais's belief, not untypical for the age, that the cause of all disease was inflammation, and since inflammation was thought to be nothing more than an excessive accumulation of blood, the prodigious use of the leech promised the best cure.

And prodigious that use was. Because of Broussais's enormous prestige, the number of leeches used in France jumped from 3 million in 1824 to 41.5 million in 1833. Physicians throughout Europe and America soon followed suit, dressing patients in so many leeches they were sometimes described as wearing glistening "coats of mail." The treatment became so fashionable it inspired a line of clothing decorated with embroidered leeches. Even traditional healers in far-flung areas of the world fell under the Western influence. Using small indigenous leeches, doctors in nineteenth-century Japan borrowed the tools and techniques of European medicine.

By the mid-nineteenth century the "inflammatory" conditions requiring treatment with leeches were legion. For headache, leeches were applied across the temples. For earache, they were applied either behind or actually in the ear. For conjunctivitis or pinkeye, they were placed within the nostril adjacent to the affected eye. For hemorrhoids and other disturbances of the bowel, leeches were set upon the anus. Leeches were also recommended for internal use, as in the abscess of a tooth. This called for the kind of logistical cleverness suggested by one Australian dentist in 1864. No need to fear that the slimy creature might wander down the throat, he pointed out, since "it can easily be held by the tail in the corner of a towel until it has fairly filled itself, or if the patient is excessively timid, a needleful of double thread can be run through the tail and tied in a loop to pass the finger through." These same precautions pertained when the leech was placed in the back of the throat to treat bronchitis and laryngitis or well within the vaginal cavity to treat uterine complaints.

Despite — or, more likely, because of — such intimate physical associations, many people had difficulty overcoming their antipathy for leeches. As one outspoken critic wrote in 1869, "The appearance of the animal is repulsive and disgusting, and delicate and sensitive persons find it difficult to overcome their repugnance to contact with the cold and slimy reptile [*sic*]." This was certainly the experience of Queen Victoria's eldest daughter, who was married to the crown prince of Prussia. When she sprained her ankle in the first months after her arrival in Berlin in 1858, the German doctors insisted on applying leeches to bring down the swelling: "Horrid slimy cold things slipping about . . . ," the princess wrote to her mother. They sickened her and made her faint.

Even setting aside repulsiveness, leeches were not without problems. Like maggots, they had a tendency to crawl out of reach. They would not always bite. And they left a tiny wound that continued to bleed for hours and ooze for days; on rare occasions the hemorrhage could not be stopped. Nonetheless, the slimy creatures were so in tune with medical theory that they became the "aspirin of the day," an appellation less ludicrous than it seems. As we know from the last chapter, bloodletting generally relieved fever and reduced certain pains and swellings, so that leeches may indeed have had an effect upon the body not unlike that of aspirin. They were certainly used as often. As a result, by the last half of the nineteenth century leeches were overcollected in the wild almost to the point of extinction. In Great Britain they were no longer to be found. Indigenous populations in France, Germany, and the United States also declined, forcing these countries to rely on imports and placing great strain on the swamps of Hungary and the Balkans. France alone purchased from abroad more than a billion leeches over the course of the century.

Medicinal use of the leech slackened by the end of the 1800s as the natural resource dwindled and as venesection as an all-purpose cure slowly expired. However, in certain reservoirs of medical tradition and medical need, physicians and other healers remained firmly attached to *Hirudo medicinalis* well into the twentieth century. Pharmacists serving certain immigrant sections of New York and Boston provided leeches and leeching expertise through the 1920s for common complaints such as black eyes. The same services could be found even in the 1950s in Cleveland.

Given the growing reluctance of early twentieth-century doctors to let blood, we might expect leeching to have been confined at this time to folk medicine, but it was not. In the 1940s physicians in Australia and in France were still using leeches to treat acute glaucoma, a disease caused by abnormally high fluid pressure within the eyeball. From 1900 to 1950 European and even American doctors still turned to leeches for what they believed to be inflammatory conditions in polio, for postoperative treatment of cancer, for bloodletting in hypertensive diseases, for the "decongestion" of inflamed deep-lying organs, for reducing the swelling of acute pericarditis, an inflammation of the membranous sac enclosing the heart, and for resolving lower-extremity thrombophlebitis, an inflammation of a vein at the site of blood clot formation.

Most of this leeching was done in Russia, Yugoslavia, Germany, Spain, France, Australia, and the countries of South America. Indeed, in certain very conservative regions of eastern and Asian Europe, leeching for hypertension, coronary and rheumatic heart disease, and chronic pulmonary disease continues today. In Great Britain and the United States the "disgusting practice" was entirely abandoned by midcentury. Remaining receptive to the past, however, can be as daring in medicine as looking forward. Thus it was from a European backwater that there sprang the innovative revival of leeching in plastic surgery.

In 1960 two Yugoslavian surgeons, M. Derganc and F. Zdravic, published an article in the *British Journal of Plastic Surgery* describing their use of leeches to relieve the venous congestion of skin transplants. With revealing candor, these two pioneers acknowledged that they got the idea from a French text of 1836. They were receptive to such an old technique because the leech was still very much a part of the eastern European medical armamentarium. Because leeching was no longer taken seriously as a medical tool in the West, however, almost total silence greeted the publication of the Yugoslavians' groundbreaking paper. Nevertheless, their innovation worked its way toward general acceptance. Within ten years their techniques were being carefully repeated in microsurgical procedures, first in France, then in Great Britain and the United States. By the 1980s the "slimy worm" had squirmed back into the forefront of medicine.

In fact, leeching has grown prodigiously since Derganc and Zdravic first tried it in 1960. From the mid-1970s to the present, leeches have been used in tissue transplants after skin loss, in breast reconstruction after mastectomy, in the treatment of periorbital hematomas, or severe black eyes, in the reduction of postoperative swelling, and in the reattachment of severed fingers, scalps, ears, lips, and penises when surgical repair of veins is incomplete or impossible. In 1988 alone more than 10,000 leeches were sold for medicinal purposes in the United States — nowhere near the millions sold in France a century and a half ago, but not an insignificant number.

The pairing of an ancient technique with modern medical endeavors has not come without controversy. Early in the past decade medical practitioners and scientists expressed great concerns about the availability of leeches, their acceptability to the patient as well as the surgeon, their medical effectiveness, and the risk of infection from their use. All of these issues have now been well resolved. Leech farms such as Roy T. Sawyer's Biopharm in Wales supply *Hirudo medicinalis* worldwide. Physicians and patients learn to tolerate leeches as easily as they do maggots. Simple antiseptic procedures ensure that leeches do not contaminate wounds. And, perhaps most important, the use of leeches significantly improves rates of salvage for transplanted or replanted tissues, especially when venous repair is technically impossible. No alternative therapy, no mechanical decongestant yet invented, can beat the leech in the last-chance effort to save tissue dying of venous congestion. In fact, if the leech sucks half-heartedly or refuses to bite at all, it is almost certain that the tissue replant cannot be salvaged by any means.

When all is said and done, we cannot do without the "horrid things" in a wide range of plastic-surgery procedures. But that is not the whole of it. Leeches have also been resurrected in the modern treatment of heart disease — though in a form more appropriate to technology-based medicine — because, in fact, the leech is more than just a lancet. Down through the ages practitioners have observed that leech bites continued to bleed long past the time when a similar cut by a knife would have ceased flowing. In the 1880s the British scientist John B. Haycraft resolved to find out why as part of his work on the physiology of blood. After much research in England and Germany, he discovered an anticoagulant substance in leech saliva that later became known as hirudin.

Haycraft was never able to isolate that active substance, but others in following decades were somewhat more successful. A purified extract of leech heads allowed scientists to analyze the blood-clotting process in the early 1900s and facilitated, too, the initial development of the artificial kidney machine in 1914. Cleansing the blood of harmful waste products by mechanical means necessarily required an anticoagulant agent. Enthusiasm for further clinical development of leech extract was dampened, however, by the finding that animals repeatedly exposed to leech extract became resistant to its anticoagulant effects. In addition, hirudin sometimes caused toxic allergic reactions due, at least some researchers thought, to impurities in its preparation. The medical use of leech saliva was stymied by repeated failure in the first five decades of this century to isolate hirudin in pure form.

The development of two other anticoagulants during this period saw considerably more progress. Heparin, an anticoagulant discovered in liver extracts, became available by the 1930s and contributed directly to the clinical success of the artificial kidney machine. During the 1940s yet another anticoagulant, warfarin, was isolated from sweet clover mold. It was subsequently marketed for human use as Coumadin in the 1950s. The clinical use of both these anticoagulants was well established by the time a German researcher named F. Markwardt finally succeeded in separating pure hirudin from leech saliva in 1955. However, little effort was made thereafter to develop pure hirudin as a medical anticoagulant. The thousands of leeches required to produce sufficient hirudin for research and therapeutic purposes made this next to impossible. Not until 1986 were biotechnologists able to genetically engineer a recombinant hirudin that mimics the clot-blocking ability of natural hirudin and does not depend on leeches for manufacture.

Recombinant hirudin promises to be of great use in the fight against disease of the coronary arteries, the two main vessels that feed the heart. These arteries can become narrowed by fatty deposits, causing a serious disruption in blood flow that results in heart attack. To restore the blood flow surgeons have developed a technique known as angioplasty in which they snake a catheter up these clogged arteries and inflate a small balloon that compresses the fatty deposits. Unfortunately, the procedure can damage the vessel wall and result in the formation of blood clots, which are especially lethal in coronary arteries. To minimize the risk of blood clotting after angioplasty, physicians prescribe heparin, but the drug sometimes fails.

Enter recombinant hirudin. Unlike heparin, which acts indirectly to inhibit clot formation, hirudin directly blocks the clotting itself, performing ten times better than heparin under experimental conditions. Indeed, hirudin is expected to play an important role, not only in cardiovascular surgery but in the treatment of blood disorders such as disseminated intravascular coagulation (DIC), characterized by a general and fatal coagulation of the blood; in hemodialysis, when the blood is purified of harmful waste products by an artificial kidney machine; and in the treatment of thromboses, or blood-clotting events, such as occur in unstable angina and heart attack. As with all new drugs, however, researchers are proceeding with caution; it will be some time before recombinant hirudin can be marketed for human use.

If hirudin were all that *Hirudo medicinalis* had to offer, it would be enough to justify protecting the endangered species from the survival pressures created by loss of habitat and renewed scientific and medical interest. And thanks to genetic engineers who can now produce recombinant hirudin in sufficient amounts, we fortunately need not bite the hand that feeds us such extraordinary medicine. But the medicinal leech also carries other active substances, including a vasodilator, which causes blood vessels to open; an enzyme called hyaluronidase, which increases the permeability of leech saliva through human tissue and also exhibits antibiotic properties; and finally, many scientists suspect, an anesthetic that numbs the leech's bite.

Altogether, these substances explain why *Hirudo medicinalis* works so well in the replantation of fingers or scalps. Leeches remove stagnant blood and at the same time inject anticoagulating, vasodilating, and antibiotic substances that work to maintain a healing circulation of the blood. Because of the striking effects of leeches in plastic surgery and because of the potential benefits in treating cardiovascular disease, each of these substances begs investigation for medical use. To this end, leech farms such as Sawyer's Biopharm harvest hirudin, hyaluronidase, and other leech products as well as the live animals themselves.

The *Hirudo* family has even more to offer. Some 650 species of bloodsucking leeches harbor a "living pharmacopoeia" of substances, which may affect human blood in different ways and provide distinct therapeutic tools. With this expectation in mind, scientists went in search of the long-lost Amazonian leech *Haementeria ghilianii* in 1977. Once found, generations of the creature were bred in an American laboratory until sufficient amounts of saliva could be obtained. Analysis revealed an enzyme subsequently named hementin that breaks up blood clots during or after formation, making it a potentially significant addition to treatment for cardiovascular disease. Salivary extract from this same leech may also be useful in preventing the metastasis of certain cancers.

The development of leech-substance drugs and the use of live leeches in plastic surgery, both at the forefront of medicine today, can be interpreted as a belated "hats off" to centuries of traditional leeching. For thousands of years the nimble little phlebotomists have been put to work on a wide variety of ailments, not all of which responded to the letting of blood or even the local effects of anticoagulation or vasodilation. But we can now grant that some injuries and some diseases were assuredly helped and healed by the application of leeches, including conditions as diverse as hematomas and hypertension. In the first instance, local bloodletting can reduce uncomfortable swelling; in the second, it can reduce dangerously high blood pressures. The leech shines best, however, when a combination of bloodletting and blood thinning is called for. Such was the case in the past when leeches were used to treat thrombophlebitis, since they not only removed congested blood but dispersed the clotted blood that caused the initial irritation. In this category, too, falls our very modern dependence on leeches in plastic surgery to facilitate the circulation of blood through transplanted tissues.

Hirudo truly is a timeless hero, whose bloodsucking ways save limbs and lives and even tresses.

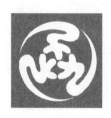

8.
LAUDABLE PUS

Many years ago, Carrel, in studying the healing
of open wounds, found that wounds "inoculated
with various dilutions of a 24-hour culture of
staphylococci in bouillon" healed faster than did
similar wounds protected from the environment by
a dressing. . . . Botsford [similarly] . . . concluded:
"It would appear that a mild wound infection
has a favorable effect on wound tensile strength,"
confirmation of our finding of enhanced healing
brought on by infection.

> — Arturo Tenorio, M.D.; Karl Jindrak, M.D.;
> Matei Weiner, M.S.; Ernesto Bella, M.S.;
> and Irving F. Enquist, M.D., 1976

F OR A SHORT TIME in 1939 the veterinarian James Herriot took over a small, very poor animal clinic in Yorkshire, England. The lack of equipment and drugs, such as the newly discovered sulfanilamides, was of little consequence for most veterinary problems. One day, however, a couple carried in a dog with a back leg so damaged — skin and muscle torn away, ligaments severed, bones broken — that Herriot sorely regretted his lack of medical materials. He ransacked the surgery shelves, finding nothing useful but a small vial of anesthetic. Then he happened on a box of plaster-of-Paris bandages and "something seemed to click." The Spanish Civil War had just ended, and Herriot recalled that "in the chaos of the later stages there had been no proper medicaments to treat the terrible wounds. They had often been encased in plaster and left, in the grim phrase, to 'stew in their own juice.' . . . I grabbed the bandages. I knew what I was going to do."

Herriot anesthetized the dog, set the broken bones, sewed up torn muscles and ligaments, and covered the leg in plaster bandaging, forming a hard cast. That was it. No modern antiseptics, no special drugs. Just a plaster cast.

A week later he saw the dog again. The once stone-hard cast, now soft and sodden with pus, exuded a sickening smell of putrefaction. Pus, of course, is formed when foreign materials or organisms contaminate a wound. The body's immune system responds to the contamination with an increase in white blood cells, or leukocytes, which engulf the foreign matter. These cells, along with tissue debris and invading microorganisms, are flushed within a serum that oozes at the site of injury. As these materials are exuded, they putrefy. Knowing this, Herriot's first response to the pus-filled cast was dismay.

"Gangrene," he thought, and steeled himself for the black and rotten flesh he expected to find under the plaster bandaging. To his immense surprise, there was no gangrene, there was almost no infection of any sort! Most of the dog's wounds had begun to heal, and to heal well. In 1987 he wrote, "How lucky I was that in those days the Spanish Civil War was still fresh in my memory. I would never have dared to encase Kim's leg in plaster if I had not read of the miraculous recoveries of the soldiers whose terrible wounds had no other means of treatment. . . . If that dog came into our surgery today, with all our antibiotics and equipment to hand I could not possibly hope that the mangled limb would heal more perfectly. The ancient surgeons used to talk about 'laudable pus.' It means something to me now."

Herriot's story is, of course, a medical confession. For every advance in modern medicine over the past fifty or even a hundred years, there is also a retreat — a technique lost, a therapy abandoned, a truth disparaged. "Laudable pus" is all of these. In its Latin form the phrase "pus bonum et laudabile" dates back to the early 1300s; the English expression, meaning commendable or healthy pus, was first used in 1420. The concept, however, is much older. The observation that pus was a natural part of wound healing had probably been made for thousands of years before the Greeks set it down in writing as a therapeutic principle. For another 1700 years the link between pus and healing held sway in Western medicine. Actual wound care, however, altered considerably during this time. The Greeks advocated the careful cleansing of wounds and the use of salves to slough off dying tissue and reduce inflammation. They recognized that pus formation could be beneficial, but they did not go out of their way to induce it in uninfected wounds.

By the Middle Ages, however, the idea that pus was *necessary* to healing had became paramount. Salves were chosen for their irritating, contaminating effects, to make the injury produce as much pus as possible. In following centuries, physicians worked with this principle in mind. When, in the mid-1500s, the military surgeon Ambroise Paré refused to treat injuries with boiling oil, he did not dispute the need for pus formation. Rather, he advocated other salves and other methods, such as the enlargement of wounds to establish drainage and "let out the sanious [bloody] pus."

Indeed, the presence of pus in wounds was almost a given until Lister introduced antiseptics to combat bacterial contamination in the mid-nineteenth century. When infection was inhibited or overcome by the use of carbolic acid or other chemicals, the body's immune defense was cut short; there was little or no pus formation. For Lister and his followers in the twentieth century, the presence of pus indicated inadequate chemical cleansing of the surgeon's tools and hands and, ultimately, of the wounded tissues themselves.

After Lister, pus was seen as an indicator of infection rather than healing. No wonder Herriot looked on that suppurating wound with trepidation! Decades of training had declared that sepsis — pus — was a failure of medical technique. The subsequent discovery of antibiotics during the 1940s made its presence even more blamable, since wounds could now be sterilized from within the body as well as from without. Today "pernicious pus" sums up the prevailing attitude. The very idea of laudable pus seems synonymous with bad, even willfully wrong-minded, medicine.

Before we consign that idea to the junk heap of medical history, however, we would do well to investigate our own immediate past. As recently as the early 1940s, just before antibiotics became widely available, pus was still considered in some medical circles an acceptable consequence of wound treatment — and not just for dogs. Aseptic technique had improved upon traditional methods but required more materials, labor, and time. When resources were strained by war or economic depression, expensive therapies were often set aside in favor of older, more expedient forms of wound care. Herriot's memoir makes the point twice: surgeons in the Spanish Civil War, and after them the English veterinarian, labored to heal in the absence of sophisticated materials and drugs. And they succeeded.

But the full story of laudable pus in the twentieth century begins with World War I. New weapons of destruction and the unprecedented conditions of trench warfare created problems the medical community had never seen before. Machine guns and exploding shells caused deep, jagged wounds, nearly all of which were contaminated with tetanus and gas gangrene — a consequence, many thought, of the manured muds of France and Flanders. The soldiers' fevers spiked, pulse rates were rapid and weak, and their dressings oozed with pus. Men died, not from their injuries but from infection.

The military physician's first response was to combat lethal bacteria with increasing amounts of antiseptic, often changing dressings several times a day. The antiseptic regimen was, in fact, taken to an extreme. In a field ambulance near Compiègne the brilliant medical scientist Alexis Carrel began experimenting with the continuous irrigation of wounds with hypochlorite. Thus World War I occasioned the first and also the last great test of the antiseptic method. By the middle of the war, however, a few lone voices were raised in dissent. Repeated antiseptic cleansing was time-consuming, costly, and excruciatingly painful for the patient.

Some field surgeons at their wits' end found that when wounds were surgically cleaned and dressed and left alone for at least a week, the patient's fever dropped, his pulse slowed, and he was able to rest undisturbed. After a few days, according to one of these surgeons, the outer bandaging was likely to become "soaked with purulent discharge." On the whole, this was considered an encouraging sign because it indicated both the absolutely critical drainage of pus away from the wound and its plentiful formation. The whole point of leaving the injury alone was in fact to permit, as another surgeon put it, "on a rising tide the swarm of leukocytes into the wound." When, finally, the pus-sodden inner dressing was removed, it came away easily and painlessly. The wound, more often than not, revealed healthy granulation tissue.

So convincing was this course of "closed" treatment to some hitherto skeptical military surgeons that they were ready to "throw all the antiseptics into the sea." This rejection of antiseptic cleansing within the wound was confirmed by a laboratory experiment not far from the front. Two British scientists, Almroth Wright and Alexander Fleming, proved in a series of classic experiments that antiseptics could not prevent or reduce infection in ragged, deep, and dirty wounds even in the best of circumstances. Wright and Fleming "discovered" what other surgeons were learning in the field, that it was the unobstructed draining of discharge, rather than any chemical wash, that helped forestall gross infection in the wound. No chemicals, no daily dressings, Wright argued. "The leucocyte is the best antiseptic."

Despite Wright's role as colonel in the British Army Medical Service, most surgeons did not relinquish "the prejudice against the formation of pus," as one proselyte of closed wound dressing complained. Nor did they readily give up the chemical methods painstakingly achieved since Lister's time. At Carrel's hospital, a mere eight miles back from the frontlines, physicians practiced rigorous antiseptic technique and "there was not a drop of pus," they claimed. By war's end, there were two camps: those who believed in antiseptic intervention and those who did not. No one quarreled, however, with the need to rest both soft-tissue wounds and bone fractures by securing them as firmly and as rigidly as possible in splints and plaster strapping. This principle, coupled with a belief in laudable pus, soon led to yet another advance in the closed method of wound care.

By 1921 H. Winnett Orr, an American lieutenant colonel back from the war, was immobilizing simple and compound fractures in plaster-of-Paris casts that provided proper alignment and extension. The method, which soon carried his name, emphasized "dependence on natural agents in healing." Although openings were left in the cast to facilitate the changing of outer, soiled dressings, Orr vigorously rejected the frequent application of antiseptics and the changing of inner dressings. After surgically cleaning and packing the wound with sterile Vaseline gauze, which served to draw pus and blood to outer dressings, the compound fracture was secured in plaster of Paris and left as long as possible, anywhere from several weeks to two months.

The Orr method was neither original nor new; infrequent dressing of wounds had had its advocates in the nineteenth century. Moreover, a method of plaster casting very similar to Orr's and dating back to the Franco-Prussian War of 1870 was still being taught in the early 1900s in Lyon, France. On the eve of World War I a few French practitioners even proposed a renewal of that traditional treatment. At the time their suggestion went unheeded, but by the 1920s and '30s, other surgeons besides Orr were reviving the practice in the United States, Austria, and France.

With the outbreak of civil war in Spain the method came into its own under the aegis of the Spanish surgeon J. Trueta. Trueta kept detailed records of his work at a base hospital in Barcelona, thereby turning three years of catastrophe into a mass clinical trial. He treated more than one thousand casualties with remarkable results. Bone and tissue fought off deadly infections, such as gas gangrene, in all but a couple of instances. Shattered arms and legs healed whole. Only six amputations were performed. Joints regained satisfactory function and mobility in three out of four cases.

All this, Trueta later argued, was due to a method especially well suited to wartime conditions. Plaster-cast encasement required few supplies and could be quickly performed, sometimes within minutes of the injury, on large numbers of people. Moreover, it allowed the immediate evacuation of wounded soldiers and civilians with a minimum of postoperative attention. French doctors complained about the stinking plasters and pus-filled wounds of the Spanish evacuees who flooded France in early 1939, but the truth was that many of the injured had traveled for days and sometimes weeks in those casts to reach safety. Closed plaster encasement saved their lives.

Just how the Orr method worked no one knew for sure. Trueta believed that immobilization constrained the flow of lymph and thus the spread of bacteria. But the most important factor, he argued, without which even immobilization would fail, was the prompt and thorough debridement of the wound, a procedure that had been gaining in importance since World War I. Best performed within six to eight hours of injury, debridement entailed the removal of all foreign matter, such as bits of shell or clothing, and the excision of all dead or dying tissue within and around the wound. Trueta not only refined this surgical preparation of the wound, he eliminated openings in the cast. Good drainage was established by the application of sterile gauze, which drew blood and pus away from the injury and disbursed them through the plaster. In the case of advanced infection, rubber tubes were also placed to further drainage from the wound. Some surgeons working in Spain had access to the new sulfonamide drugs developed in the mid-1930s to combat infection, and they sprinkled these over the injured tissue before dressing. But for Trueta and many others, plaster-encased wounds were truly healed by "the natural defenses of the body." This, then, was the controversial, apparently counterintuitive treatment that James

Herriot so vividly remembered in 1939. And to his amazement and relief, it worked, even without the sulfa drugs.

When World II broke out in earnest, the massive wounds caused by aerial bombs and shrapnel became not just a Spanish problem, but a European one. Many British surgeons, even those who had harbored "a deep-seated prejudice against the closed method of treating . . . wounded limbs," finally accepted plaster encasement as a "notable advance in treatment" no longer "on its trial." The Orr method was not without serious drawbacks, however, chief among them its characteristic pus. Bacteria passed with the pus through the plaster, creating a contamination hazard for uninfected patients in the hospital wards. But more noisome than this was the offensive smell that emanated after a day or two from the casts. Fresh pus usually did not smell bad; pus decaying in the plaster did, and it steadily worsened as time went by. In good weather, the wounded spent almost all of their time outdoors — with good reason. When, because of weather or blackout it was necessary to remain inside, "the trouble was a very real one." A few stalwart surgeons, including Trueta, argued that the smell had useful clinical significance. A truly bad odor suggested inadequate drainage of the wound or even the presence of necrotic tissue. But for most doctors and patients the issue was one of kind, not degree. Herriot found the smell of one pus-filled cast nearly unbearable. Imagine the smell of dozens and hundreds of these "stink plasters" in one room!

It comes as no surprise that despite the effectiveness of closed plaster encasement and the "poultice of pus," as one British surgeon called it, medical workers eagerly seized upon penicillin when it was finally made available in 1943. Fleming's antibiotic proved far more effective against infectious bacteria than any of the antiseptics or any of the sulfa drugs. Surgeons at the front, including the newly arrived Americans, continued to debride wounds and splint them. In addition they administered penicillin, either locally or systemically. By the time the injured reached permanent hospitals, their wounds were usually well on the way to recovery. Surgeons were able to suture without fear of further infection. Convalescence was cut in half. There was no messy plaster dressing, no contamination hazard, and no smell. A new era of wound treatment had begun, and with it a new revulsion for pus.

We must not make the mistake, however, of thinking that the old era came to an abrupt and absolute end. Indeed, laudable pus is still with us today. Danish physicians actually used the term in a medical journal a scant four years ago. They meant simply to draw the same distinction that their predecessors had. Watery, brown, foul-smelling discharge is associated with lethal systemic infections. Thick, creamy pus, which means the infection is localized, is a good sign — laudable. But laudable pus remains more than a viable definition. The concept itself, inasmuch as it postulates an association between wound irritation and wound healing, was and still is the focus of much ongoing research.

In the days before microscopes, germ theory, and scientific technique, observable laudable pus would necessarily have been the first sign of eventual healing. This association of pus with recovery made sense so long as injury was accompanied almost inevitably by infection. Yet once it became possible to inhibit infection by destroying pus-forming bacteria, the relationship between pus and healing was called into question. Wounds treated with antiseptics seemed to heal much more rapidly than grossly infected wounds, at least under certain stringent conditions. And those treated with antibiotics certainly healed more rapidly. At the same time, our knowledge of each stage of the inflammatory process became ever more detailed on the cellular level, and so did our ability to detect and analyze the earliest effects of bacterial infection at the wound site. Quite unexpectedly, researchers found at this level that some infection actually enhanced healing.

Perhaps the starting point in this line of research is Almroth Wright's work on the role of leukocytes in wound healing. His efforts to delineate the optimal conditions for these white blood cells — which in large concentrations make the discharge from a wound look white — has been called the first scientific evidence in support of laudable pus. In quite disparate work, two other well-known researchers subsequently postulated that infection and other sorts of inflammation actually stimulated the tissue-repair processes of wound healing. In 1921 Alexis Carrel reported that wounds protected from chemical, bacterial, or physical irritation did not heal as quickly as wounds dressed with standard antiseptics. Conversely, wounds exposed to chemicals or bacteria healed *more* quickly. Twenty-five years later Francis Peyton Rous realized that skin grafts "took" best when both the transferred skin and the tissue bed were in an optimally inflamed state.

A few studies in the 1940s and '50s confirmed that mild wound infection strengthened tissue by stimulating the inflammatory reaction that resulted in its formation. In these early years of antibiotic therapy nobody seemed very interested, but in the late 1970s the concept was "rediscovered" with more sophisticated techniques. In a series of interrelated experiments a group of researchers demonstrated that observable infection did in fact increase the rate of healing, as measured primarily by tissue strength determined in experiments performed in vitro, outside the living body.

These findings were disputed almost at once by other scientists investigating different kinds of wounds and different strains and concentrations of bacteria. Some rejected the link between observable infection and healing altogether. Others insisted that the benefits to healing depended upon contamination that could not be detected by the naked eye. Research in the late 1980s confirmed that the introduction of pathogenic and even non-pathogenic bacteria *in very small amounts* into the experimental wounds of laboratory rats did enhance immune response, but the magnitude of the effect depended somewhat on the type of bacteria. Such irritation shortened the period of healing by attracting white blood cells to the site of injury, increasing blood and serum flow, and stimulating the growth of new tissue.

In these latest experiments, enhanced immune response fell just short of observable pus formation — indeed, researchers found that the macroscopic appearance of pus delayed healing.

Nevertheless, they suggested that wound treatment in the future may include the controlled irritation of injured tissue with bacterial components. This kind of minute bacterial irritation may explain a recent observation that cleaning wounds with tap water instead of sterile saline solution cut the observable infection rate in half. Moreover, we already irritate wounds chemically every time we use iodine or Mercurochrome or hydrogen peroxide. These substances draw white blood cells in amounts just short of observable pus into injured tissue and thus promote healing.

We "know better" than to induce uncontrolled infection in a wound as our forebears often did, yet the principle of wound irritation is a sound one. With standard antibiotics beginning to lose effectiveness, the prospect of promoting health by means of controlled or benign infection begins once again to look promising. Just recently some researchers suggested that certain types of bacteria and yeast be used to combat diarrheal and vaginal infections. As the scientists acknowledged, this approach is very like the traditional practice of making poultices from moldy bread or fermented milk. Our ancestors healed wounds by manipulating bacterial infection in a gross and clumsy way. They did not have the knowledge or technique to control bacterial irritation at the microscopic level. Increasingly we do; we are able in many cases to induce a "laudable irritation" without the pus. What separates our techniques from those of the past is only a matter of degree.

It is time we recognize the bonus in laudable pus. Our horror of suppuration is not a natural revulsion, it is a modern squeamishness resulting almost wholly from our dependence upon effective antibiotics. Yet, whether wound management depends on macroscopic or microscopic inflammation, the intent across the centuries has always been the same — to promote healing. Techniques based upon observable infection were not deliberately or necessarily wrong-minded. Laudable pus, far from being an ancient stupidity, remained a viable medical concept of wound care well into World War II. In the absence of antibiotics and stringent antiseptic care, a "poultice of pus" allowed twentieth-century men like Orr and Trueta and Herriot to heal horrendous wounds. The principle behind that care, that local infection stimulates immune response and wound repair, is still with us today.

People may dress wounds with more or with less sophistication, but it is nature that heals them.

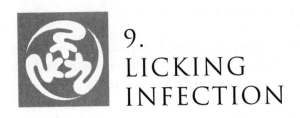

9.
LICKING
INFECTION

Licking one's wounds may be more than metaphor.
— I. D. Mandel, D.D.S., 1987

THE MOVIE *Quest for Fire* has a number of gut-wrenching scenes, one of which involves a caveman who has been badly mauled by a bear. He survives the encounter with huge bite and claw wounds all over his body. Subsequent scenes show his clansmen licking his cuts and scabs. Although the film is obviously fictitious, many of its premises, including this one, are derived from reasonable assumptions about how our ancestors behaved as we evolved from apelike creatures into human beings. Many of our nearest animal relatives, including all of the great apes, lick their own wounds and those of their close relatives with therapeutic results, and it is difficult to see why the same should not have been true for early man.

The licking of human wounds has been amply recorded in much more recent times. A famous instance involved Niccolò Fontana, one of the greatest mathematicians of the Italian Renaissance, who is better known to history as Tartaglia, the Stammerer. He received his nickname as a result of a horrible childhood injury inflicted by a French soldier during an attack on his hometown in 1512. Tartaglia's face was slashed by the soldier's sword, resulting in a lifelong speech impediment. According to legend, apparently reasonably well corroborated, Tartaglia survived only because a faithful dog licked his wound religiously, keeping it clean and helping it to heal.

Similar stories pepper the legends of pioneers who opened up the Americas during the seventeenth and eighteenth centuries. American Indians were sometimes reported to present a wound to their dogs for licking, and even, according to one story, to such an unlikely caregiver as a female moose! In most historical cases human wounds were licked by animals, but reliable sources document that Indians themselves sucked on wounds caused by arrows and bullets until the blood stopped flowing, in the process undoubtedly introducing saliva into injured tissue. American and European physicians who witnessed these treatments almost universally commented that the results of Indian wound therapy were far superior to their own.

And salivating at wounds continues to this day. "Dog Licks Man" is the title of a 1970 account by Lindsay Verrier, a resident of Fiji in the South Pacific. Although it sounds like a *National Enquirer* headline, Verrier's article appeared in the British medical journal *The Lancet*. Verrier recounted awakening from a nap one day to find his dog licking a scrape on his leg. "To my surprise, the operation was painless," he recalled, and the wound healed quickly and well. In consequence he offered his dog a second scrape some time later, with equally good results. "I mentioned this to a Fijian friend, who told me that in the villages, when lads got sores on their legs from fishing, gardening, and so on, the old men advised them to let the dogs lick them, so as to heal them quickly."

Many other people apparently allow their pets to lick their cuts and scrapes, too; how many it is impossible to know, but some cases have caught the attention of physicians over the last ten years because they involved complications. In Cleveland, Ohio, a diabetic patient suffering from ulceration of the foot allowed her dog to lick the sore. In Denmark several men with leg ulcers allowed their dogs to lick their wounds, as did a man in New York suffering from chronic kidney failure. In Nantes, France, a woman with sores associated with a rare blood disease was similarly licked by her dog. Dogs have also reportedly licked the wounds and abrasions of children. Since the number of reports that actually enter the medical literature is only a small fraction of any set of medical occurrences, we can assume that these cases are but the tip of an iceberg obscured by an ocean of denial. In most of these cases the outcome is good, so physicians need never be the wiser.

Our modern "civilized" sensibilities may shudder at the thought, but we suspect that most of us can remember licking our cuts and scrapes to get the blood off, and even eating — yes, eating! — some of our scabs when we were children. But who wants to admit that as a grown-up — and to a doctor! The trouble is, our adult reluctance to lick our wounds or have them licked ignores some pretty basic physiological drives. Blood has the sort of salty-sweet flavor that most of us find appealing. Fresh pus tastes sweet, too — a fact that was undoubtedly noted in prehistory and certainly put in writing by 1794, when John Hunter wrote his *Treatise on the Blood, Inflammation and Gunshot Wounds*. Our taste buds, at least, are not averse to wound care. No wonder that animals and children naturally lick their wounds.

Squeamishness has to be carefully taught, and in our culture it most definitely is. Trained as we are to avoid all possible causes of infection, by the time we are adults, having a dog, let alone a friend, lick our wounds strikes us as unsanitary and unseemly. Certainly, no animal book lists wound licking as a pet prerogative. Saliva can carry a wide range of pathogenic organisms that no one would knowingly want to introduce under the skin, including various types of streptococci, staphylococci, a relative of the cholera bacillus called *Pasteurella multocida,* and rabies. In fact, several medical cases have been reported of very ill or immune-suppressed individuals contracting opportunistic infections — that is, infections from organisms that are not disease-causing in healthy individuals — when pets licked their open sores. So the risk is real, if small. In general, however, most human saliva does not contain enough of these germs to be harmful, and most of the germs that populate a dog's mouth are probably even less of a risk.

This may be news to many whose cultural conditioning is thorough. The very notion that wound licking might benefit the licked individual, that it might, in fact, be a natural survival mechanism, has become a topic of medical research only within the last fifteen years. Logically, most of the earliest work focused on the effect that licking wounds has on the rate of healing in animals such as mice, rats, and dogs. It was found that saliva almost invariably speeded healing dramatically while simultaneously decreasing the probability of infection. In all of these studies, the animals licked themselves, so the possibility of infection from another animal was unlikely.

Next on the research agenda was the effect of human saliva on wounds of the oral cavity. As most of us have probably observed without thinking about it, cuts in the mouth heal quickly. You bite your lip or the inside of your cheek so deeply that it bleeds, yet within seconds the bleeding usually stops; a few hours later, although it still hurts, there is no scab and the sore is already healing. Moreover, mouth infections from such cuts are extremely rare, except in people with serious immune deficiencies. Odd, isn't it?

Actually, once you know what is in saliva, its wound-healing properties are anything but mysterious. As one oral surgeon has written, "Saliva possesses a multiplicity of defense systems for antibacterial warfare that the Pentagon can envy." In the first place, saliva is part of the immune system. Along with the mucus produced by membranes in the eyes, nose, throat, and other openings of the body, saliva contains a large amount of water, which functions to wash away dirt and germs. It also contains proteins with various digestive and antibiotic functions. The digestive proteins, or enzymes, include amylase, which chemically converts starches to sugar, and the proteases, which break down proteins into smaller fragments called peptides and even smaller components called amino acids. These enzymes have some limited antimicrobial action, but the other proteins in saliva have specific antiseptic and antibiotic properties. The first to be discovered was lysozyme, an enzyme that eats away the protective coating of many types of bacteria. The research that led to its discovery in 1921 was undertaken by the Scottish bacteriologist Alexander Fleming seven years prior to his better-known discovery of penicillin, for which he shared a Nobel Prize.

Fleming's discovery came about in a typically roundabout, atypically outrageous way, some time after he became aware of the work of Felix d'Hérelle and Frederick Twort on what they termed "bacteriophages." Bacteriophages, we now know, are viruses that infect and kill bacteria; hence their name: "bacteria eaters." The only two types known at the time caused diarrhea: one type was associated with human dysentery, the other with — believe it or not — diarrhea in locusts. Fleming, in his characteristically playful manner, conceived the crazy idea that if bacteriophages could cause gastrointestinal "runs," perhaps they were also responsible for "runny" noses.

Fleming, being particularly susceptible to colds as a result of a badly healed broken nose, began culturing his own nasal mucus for signs of bacteriophage. In November 1921 he succeeded in isolating what he thought was the first viral agent responsible for upper respiratory problems. It had all the right properties: it was present when he was ill, it killed a particular bacterium associated with his cold, and it was too small to see. A bit more work, however, showed that it was not a bacteriophage — among other things, it couldn't reproduce. Instead it turned out to be an enzyme present in all mucus, saliva, and tears that was capable of eating away the membranes with which some bacteria protect themselves. Fleming's mentor, the immunologist Almroth Wright, suggested that he call the new agent lysozyme: "enzyme that lyses (or breaks open)" bacteria. And so it was named.

Since Fleming's day, reports of other antibacterial agents present in saliva have continued to dribble in at a surprisingly constant rate. The salivary arsenal is now known to include mucins, fibronectin, beta-2 microglobulin, lactoferrins, salivary peroxidases, histatins, cystatins, antibodies, and other as yet unidentified agents, all with specialized capabilities.

Mucins and fibronectin appear to inactivate some microbes by directly binding them up, thereby preventing them from infecting their target cells. Lactoferrins kill iron-dependent bacteria by binding up the iron they need to survive. Peroxidases essentially convert the hydrogen peroxide produced by bacteria into bacterial poisons. Whenever it comes in contact with foreign agents, the immune system secretes antibodies and beta-2 microglobulin. Both kinds of protein have specific antimicrobial effects. One type of antibody, known as IgA, is particularly prevalent in saliva. IgA antibodies help protect against bacteria and also many viruses as well, including polio and influenza.

The most recently characterized groups of agents in saliva are the cystatins and histatins, proteins that have multiple functions. Their primary one is apparently that of building strong teeth, but both groups have antibacterial and important antifungal activity. In fact, significant efforts are being made to genetically engineer the cystatin and histatin genes into E. coli or yeasts in order to mass-produce them for therapeutic purposes. The effort is particularly worthwhile since modern medicine is woefully short of good antifungal drugs.

Among the still unidentified antimicrobial agents present in saliva, undoubtedly the most interesting is something that appears to protect people against oral infection by the human immunodeficiency virus, HIV. One speculation is that the anti-HIV agent will be found among the wide range of molecules in saliva that interfere with the proteases. This would seem to make sense, since the destructive effects of HIV depend upon a protease that has become the most recent target of pharmaceutical companies trying to stop AIDS. At the time this book is being written, protease inhibitors are the biggest news on the AIDS treatment front. Given the amount of time and money spent developing AIDS medicines, it would certainly be ironic if the kind of anti-HIV agent we need has been lurking all this time in saliva.

Saliva also contains many healing agents that speed the regrowth of tissue and closure of wounds. Perhaps the most medically significant are the growth factors. As with Fleming's discovery of lysozyme, the discovery of growth factors came about indirectly, earning both Rita Levi-Montalcini and Stanley Cohen a Nobel

Prize. During the late 1940s Levi-Montalcini was investigating ways to manipulate the development of the nervous system in chickens. She began by transplanting extra limb buds and other organs onto the thin membrane that surrounds developing chick embryos inside their eggs. These grafts sent chemical messages to the developing embryo, causing it to produce nerves connecting itself to the grafts in unexpected ways. Levi-Montalcini's object was to determine what chemical signals the nervous system uses to grow and mature as it does.

Colleagues drew her attention to a paper reporting that some types of tumor cells caused a huge proliferation of nerve tissue in chick embryos. Levi-Montalcini verified this observation and found that many normal tissues seemed to secrete the same chemical messenger but in much smaller amounts. At this point Stanley Cohen entered the picture, taking on the arduous task of isolating and identifying the chemical messenger in the tumor cells. In the process he resorted to using a preparation of snake venom, which was supposed to destroy a chemical contaminant of the tumor extract. Quite unexpectedly, he found that the venom contained more of the nerve growth factor than did the tumor!

Once the identity of nerve growth factor was established, Cohen searched for its sources in the body. To his surprise (though the venom should have provided a clue), the main source turned out to be the salivary glands. Moreover, in a partially purified batch of nerve growth factor, Cohen discovered a substance he dubbed epidermal growth factor, which specifically enhanced the growth of connective tissue and skin cells. Thus saliva turned out to be the major source of two of the key growth factors that are now known to enhance wound healing. Another, platelet-derived growth factor (PDGF), comes from blood. Others, such as glial growth factors and transforming growth factors, have now been identified as well, though not in saliva.

All of the known growth factors are currently being tested by pharmaceutical and biotechnology companies for use in wound-care products. The list of universities, hospitals, and companies currently investigating nerve growth factor and epidermal growth factor for their potential in healing is very long and includes institutions in Cuba, Japan, Switzerland, and Australia. Epidermal growth factor is being used in the treatment of external ulcers, stomach ulcers, oral ulcers, esophageal burns caused by caustic agents, surgical wounds, and thermal burns. Nerve growth factor is being tested in clinics for its ability to stop nerve loss associated with diabetic neuropathies, Alzheimer's disease, and Parkinson's disease.

Other growth factors are also undergoing clinical evaluation. For example, the Emory Wound Healing and Limb Preservation Clinic in Atlanta, Georgia, is currently conducting a trial of transforming growth factor–beta 2 for the treatment of nonhealing ulcers in diabetic patients. Chiron Corporation and Johnson and Johnson are collaborating on clinical trials of a wound-healing agent they are calling Regranex (becaplermin), a formulation containing as its active ingredient recombinantly produced human platelet-derived growth factor. And Cambridge Neuroscience is developing glial growth factor for clinical use.

Other active agents in saliva have also been developed for pharmaceutical use. For at least forty years Fleming's lysozyme has been used by eastern European countries for treating surgical wounds. The gene for histatin, the main salivary antifungal agent, has been engineered into cells that now produce "buckets of the stuff," according to one researcher. The purified protein is being tested for topical treatments of fungal infections. Soon investigators hope to introduce the cells into the salivary glands of animals as a first step toward genetically engineering greater production of the protein in AIDS patients and others with inadequate immune systems. Some researchers are even trying to produce "artificial saliva" for the use of people who, because of various medical conditions, including the autoimmune disease known as Sjögren's syndrome, are unable to produce sufficient saliva.

Perhaps such sterile "synthetic spit" may one day be used for wound care. For when all is said and done, except for the risk of contamination, everyday saliva turns out to be an excellent wound dressing. It protects injured tissue, promotes healing, usually prevents further infection, and is virtually painless. These are necessary attributes in any would-be dressing. Does this mean saliva, or its synthetic variants, will soon be at the forefront of wound care? More to the point, if the real thing is so good, should we wait for the artificial stuff? "Should we," asks Elizabeth Sherertz of the Department of Dermatology at the Bowman Gray–Wake Forest University Medical Center, "have our patients lick their wounds?" Is there, she adds irreverently, a positive side to the scathing remark surgeons make to their nervous students dripping with sweat: "Why don't you just spit into the wound?"

Not really! "In theory," Sherertz pointedly answers, "there might be benefits, but I am not sure that such a study would make it through a human experimentation committee." Not many patients would understand or consent to such experimental guidelines anyway. Of course, life sometimes alters our perceptions. If no water were available and chemical antisepsis were not a possibility, a wounded person might reasonably use a bit of spit to forestall serious infection and speed healing. In a clinical setting, however, our preference for manufactured medication over a natural remedy such as saliva is justified by the protection from cross-contamination.

So what's the point of raising tongue-in-cheek questions? They do draw serious attention to the ways in which clinical medicine can benefit from the investigation of natural therapies such as wound licking. As Sherertz points out, the development of drugs derived from salivary components is conservative but fundamentally sound. In the search for ever better wound care it makes sense to learn as much as possible from fellow creatures still licking infection the old-fashioned way.

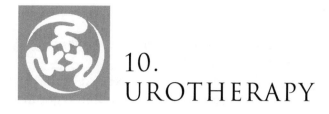

10.
UROTHERAPY

*The use of urine in the pharmacopoeia of many
ancient nations has generally been written
off in modern times. . . . Historians of medicine,
however, might have been more circumspect in such
condemnations after the classical discovery of
S. Aschheim and B. Zondek in 1927 of the presence
of large amounts of sex hormones in pregnancy
urine, and the subsequent realization that all urine,
but especially that of certain animals such as the
mare, contains these active substances. . . . This
forms a really rather extraordinary story.*

— Joseph Needham, Sc.D., and
Lu Gwi-Djen, Ph.D., 1968

DISASTERS and hopelessness lead people to try unusual and sometimes extreme therapies. People with AIDS unfortunately are prey to both. Until recently, doctors and patients faced with this disease have been largely helpless. Not surprisingly, many people with AIDS have therefore resorted to unconventional medicines in search of relief for their symptoms.

One of the more unusual practices recently came to light in *Continuum Magazine,* put out by a British "organization for long-term survivors of HIV and AIDS and people who want to be." Continuum member Phil Heath says, "Yes, I will admit, I drink my own urine. I also use it on my skin as well. This practice, which is known as Amoroli or Urine Therapy has been used as a therapy in many cultures since the dawn of time."

It is a therapy, however, that has become extremely uncommon. Heath himself had not heard of it before his illness got the better of him and his doctors in October 1992. At that point his immune system was slowly collapsing, he felt continuously unwell, and he was depressed. Worst of all, he had developed a serious outbreak of molluscum contagiosum, an infectious viral disease resulting in large, pulpy nodules filled with yellowish pus that appear most frequently on the face, neck, and shoulders. Conventional therapies not only failed to help Heath, they were time-consuming and unpleasant. "Personally I would have done almost anything to have got rid of these unsightly eruptions from my face, so I was ready for anything. It was then that a friend advised me to apply my own urine to my skin at the sight [sic] of the eruptions and, open to any suggestion which might help, I did."

Heath reports that within a few weeks his molluscum outbreak had vanished, and subsequent eruptions were both small and limited. Unfortunately, about the same time he contracted oral thrush (moniliasis), a yeast infection of the mouth and throat caused by *Candida albicans*. He also developed hairy leukoplakia, an oral infection associated with the presence of active Epstein-Barr virus (the cause of mononucleosis) in immune-suppressed people. Again, conventional medical therapies made little dent in Heath's symptoms and he grew desperate. The same friend who had advised him to wash his skin with urine also advised him to drink his urine to cure the oral infections. Lacking a viable alternative and having just experienced the positive effects of urine washing, Heath steeled himself for yet another experiment.

"I have to admit," he writes, "it is quite difficult to overcome the brainwashing of a lifetime which has taught us that our own urine is dirty . . . but, I simply got up one morning, peed into a cup and drank the lot. . . . That first batch was terrible."

Nonetheless, Heath continued to drink his urine daily, and as he did so he noticed the taste less and less. More intriguingly, he claims that not only did his oral infections disappear, but he began to sleep better, feel better, and have better blood test results. Heath now drinks not only his morning urine, but some of his urine each time he passes water. And he continues to wash with it. He's certain, despite his doctors' skepticism, that his urine therapies are helping.

Oddly, at about the same time that Heath began experimenting with urine for his AIDS-associated symptoms, a set of physicians in the United States found quite a different group of people using urine for many similar reasons. In this instance the finding was not relegated to the pages of a small-circulation newsletter but publicized in national newspapers: "RESEARCHER DISCOVERS SHOCKING CHILD-CARE PRACTICES," read the December 1988 headline from United Press International. The article, "Black Child Care Practices in the Midwest," described the findings of a team of doctors and nurses led by Dr. John Walburn, head of general pediatrics at the University of Nebraska Medical Center in Omaha.

The team had become aware that many ethnic groups prefer folk practices to conventional medical treatments and that caring for such patients required a nonjudgmental understanding of those practices. The most unusual custom that the team documented among poor midwestern blacks involved various uses of what they called "pee diapers" — that is, in the medical terminology of the paper, "diapers wet with urine but no stool." Twenty-two percent of the caregivers and mothers interviewed by the medical team used pee diapers to cleanse their babies' skin rashes; 18 percent used them to treat infantile acne or hives, and 15 percent used the diapers to wipe out an infant's mouth if it was suffering from thrush. "In fact," the team reported, "a number of care givers anecdotally related wiping their own faces with them to improve the complexion." Heath, at least, would have recognized the therapeutic intent.

People in other times and places would have, too. Neither drinking nor bathing the skin with urine are unique to people with AIDS or a few African-American mothers. Urine, like saliva, appears and reappears in the pharmacopoeias of many cultures.

One of its most widespread uses is in the treatment of wounds and sores. The Ebers Papyrus and the Hearst Medical Papyrus, both from around 1500 B.C., record a burn salve of ground gourd seeds, salt, and urine. The Ebers Papyrus even suggests that the ancient Egyptians may have used urine to cleanse burns when water was not available. One medical incantation reads:

> "Your son Horus has burned himself in the desert."
> "Is there any water here?"
> "There is no water here."
> "Water is in my mouth, a Nile is between my thighs, I have come to extinguish the fire."
> "Flow out, burn!"

Interestingly enough this ages-old therapy probably explains why, three millennia later, British officers serving in the Sahara during World War II observed Arabs urinating on the open wounds of British soldiers. At first the British were shocked and interpreted the action as gross insubordination and an offense to flag and country. Actually it was a way of cleaning and sterilizing wounds developed by people who rarely have access to plentiful water. And it is still used today. In Iran children are still taught to wash their wounds with their own urine if no fresh water is available.

Across the world in another arid region, a similar regimen was advocated by the Aztecs five hundred years ago. One of their medical texts advises the physician to wash wounds with warm, fresh urine, treat with herbs and sweet maguey sap, and, according to recent scholars, "allow the natural processes to take over unless signs of infection appear requiring repetition of the treatment." Some American Indians also used urine for regular skin care. In 1806, on their famous expedition to map the Northwest Territories, Meriwether Lewis and William Clark found a group of Indians in the Oregon area who, in Lewis's words, "have a very singular custom among them of bathing themselves all over with urine every morning." Modern readers may be relieved to know that these Indians also frequently bathed in springs and ponds.

The Hindu tradition of Ayurvedic medicine, whose texts date anywhere from 1000 B.C. to A.D. 1000, also made ample use of urine. For example, a primary medical manual known as the *Charaka Samhita* describes the ideal hospital as having among its pharmaceutical stores "oil, fat, marrow, honey, treacle, salt . . . different kinds of wines, whey, butter-milk, sour gruel of paddy or rice, and the different varieties of animal urine." The urines were used in poultices mixed with herbs to treat wounds; in plasters mixed with herbs and curds to treat fevers; and, intriguingly, as enemas to treat internal abscesses. Perhaps the most unusual use of urine was in a "soup" with milk. This soup was boiled to produce steam and directed by means of pipes onto postoperative wounds. It is not at all clear from this distant perspective why the steam — a source of heat that would stimulate blood flow and tissue regeneration — could not have been produced by water alone, but presumably the Hindu practitioners had their reasons.

The Chinese also used urine medicinally at least 2000 years ago in connection with various Taoist practices. Their texts included many references to urine's effects on sexual health, and Chhu Chhêng, a fifth-century physician, also recommended urine to stop bleeding. Somewhat later, pre-Renaissance Italians used mixed decoctions of wine and urine to remove parasitic worms infesting the ear canals. As one medical researcher sportively notes, the urine may at least have made the worms "uncomfortable."

Ancient medical practitioners also found other uses for urine. Consider the derivation of the term "diabetes mellitus," the scientific name for what we more commonly call insulin-dependent diabetes. The term originated in pre-Christian Greece. "Diabetes" comes from the Greek word meaning to pass water, and "mellitus" is from the same root word as honey. In other words, diabetes mellitus means "to pass sweet water." Now, how did Greek physicians more than 2500 years ago know that the urine passed by diabetics was sweet? Given their lack of chemical knowledge and of modern analytical techniques, there is only one possible answer: they *tasted* it. In fact, virtually all medical texts from Greek times through the early modern era advised physicians on the many ways in which the look, smell, and taste of urine revealed the health of the individual. Modern urinalysis, using chemical reactions and automated techniques, is simply a high-tech version, with the additional benefit of quantification, of what the tongue, eye, and nose of the physician have done for thousands of years.

Tasting urine is one thing. Actually imbibing it is another. And yet urine and chemicals distilled from it have been ingested as therapeutic agents since ancient times. Perhaps the oldest records concern the age-old practice of *amoroli*, which Phil Heath used in his fight against his AIDS-associated infections. This Hindu ritual involves the drinking of one's morning urine. The *Damara Tantra*, a classic Hindu text, contains the following advice: "A sensible man gets up early in the morning when three quarters of the night has passed (i.e., about 3 or 4 o'clock), faces east and passes urine. The initial and concluding flow of urine is to be discarded. The intermediate flow is to be consumed. This is the most suitable method."

The purpose of this ritual, which has equivalents in other yogic texts as well, is not clear from available sources. In traditional Indian writings, amoroli is usually associated with specific dietary restrictions (little meat, many fruits and vegetables, no drugs or alcohol), fasting, and meditation. It is possible that the combination of diet or fasting and urine ingestion promotes the meditative state. Some Hindu texts also recommend amoroli as a revitalizing technique, and the most recent Indian works have recommended it as an adjunct to therapies for "ailments ranging from skin disorders to AIDS and cancers." At least two prime ministers of India, Mahatma Gandhi and Morarji Desai, have publicly extolled the virtues of amoroli, calling urine "the water of life."

It would be a mistake, however, to think that only Hindus have swallowed urine therapy: people on every inhabited continent have done so. For chest injuries Aztec physicians prescribed ingesting urine into which "three or four lizards" had been thrown. The Kikuyu tribe in Africa have traditionally drawn blood from their cattle, mixed it with milk and cow's urine, and allowed the liquid to ferment for a few days to a soft cheeselike consistency before eating it. The Dinkas of the Nile Valley in southern Sudan make a similar mixture and also use urine (in this case from a cow) to ritually wash their hands and faces. And the ancient Romans are reported to have used urine as a mouthwash — a practice that probably did have limited antibacterial (and therefore cavity-fighting) effects. But talk about morning breath!

Urine, as well as all other bodily secretions, was a staple of folk medicines concocted in ancient China. Among other uses, urine ingestion was prescribed to treat sore throats, lung diseases, and asthma and to open clogged blood vessels in pregnant women. The most frequent and oldest use of urine by the Chinese, however, was to stimulate sexual activity. Some evidence exists that Taoists may have prescribed the drinking of urine to improve sexual performance as long ago as 200 A.D., and a continuous record of its use for this purpose exists since the fourteenth century. Most remarkably, by the eleventh century the Chinese had learned how to purify various sediments and precipitates from urine, sometimes reducing hundreds of liters of golden liquid to a few grams of pure crystalline or pearly white material. These purified, or semipurified, chemicals would then be resolubilized in other drinks to please fastidious royalty who objected to the "unclean origin" of urine itself. In perhaps one of the earliest examples of clever advertising, these urine concentrates were dispensed under the innocuous names "autumn mineral" and "autumn ice."

Seventeenth- and eighteenth-century European doctors also prescribed urine (usually from cows) for their patients. Like Chinese physicians, they found that properly identifying the material gave "the sick an idea that was false and disgusting." In a flush of genius, they invented euphemistic names such as the French *l'eau de mille fleurs* ("water of a thousand flowers"). Patients were admonished to drink "two or three glasses" of this distillation "every morning . . . for gout, the 'vapors,' etc."

For the less squeamish, distilled human urine under its own name was also prescribed for these ailments. In the case of gout, human urine was believed to cleanse the body of the injurious causes of the disease. For the vapors, a hysterical giddiness apparently common among women in early modern Europe, urine was thought to have a calming effect. A letter from Madame de Sévigné, one of the favorites of Louis XIV, to her daughter in 1685 suggests that she drank distilled urine to induce sleep: "For my vapors, I take eight drops of the essence of urine [a concentrated formulation made by boiling off some of the water from the urine of a young man who had drunk a good deal of wine], and contrary to what usually happens, it kept me from sleeping." Essence of urine was also recommended for apoplexy (stroke), epilepsy, convulsions, palsies, lethargies, and vertigos!

Both the external and the internal uses of urine raise some urgent questions. Might it actually have any beneficial therapeutic uses? Is it really wise to put it on a wound? Is it hygienic to taste or ingest urine, regardless of its medical effects? Is it really all right to use "pee diapers" therapeutically? Isn't urine full of germs and loaded with disgusting waste chemicals? Isn't it dangerous? To answer these questions we have to get up close and personal with urine itself.

The task is not as awful as it seems at first. Oddly enough, fresh urine from a healthy person or animal — one who does not have, for example, kidney disease, urinary tract infection, or sexually transmitted disease — is sterile. It contains no germs, or only the few that it picks up as it leaves the urinary tract and comes in contact with the tip of the penis or the labia. Urine just extracted from a healthy individual, therefore, usually poses no infectious threat. It follows that urinating on a wound or wiping a rash or yeast infection is quite reasonable, if no pure source of water is available. Significantly, people in the past recognized that only fresh urine would do — a wise precaution, since urine that has been standing will grow all kinds of microorganisms. Moreover, if you are going to drink urine, it should always be your own so that you avoid exposure to infection. As the Bible says: "Drink waters out of thine own cistern" — a proverb many urine drinkers like to quote.

And from their own "cisterns" some people have indeed

drunk with little or no ill effect. People without access to fresh water, stranded at sea or lost in the desert, have often resorted to drinking their own urine to keep from dying of dehydration. Whole populations have even resorted to the practice under extreme conditions. During a terrible drought in Amman, Jordan, in 1970, the Red Crescent (the Middle East's equivalent of the Red Cross) actually recommended urine drinking as a lifesaving measure. "Your children are expiring of thirst," ran the radio announcements. "We cannot help you except by telling you that you may be able to save their lives by letting them drink their own urine. It will cause them no harm!"

Just as surprising as the (generally) sterile nature of fresh urine is that its chemical contents, as bad as they can smell, are largely nontoxic and have some interesting properties that have made them widely appreciated within the pharmaceutical industry. A typical urine specimen contains about 95 percent water and 5 percent solids, although both the percentage of water and the contents of the solids vary widely between individuals and from one time to another. The solids are almost always mainly urea and sodium chloride, that is, salt. Urea is the more interesting from our perspective, for it is the primary means of excreting nitrogen from the body and plays a crucial role in permitting the kidneys to maintain the water balance of the body. Urea has so little toxicity that it would take about one hundred grams, or about three and a half ounces, of pure urea to kill an average man. Relying on that chemical fact, Princeton professor Hubert Alyea used to introduce the subject of organic chemistry in the 1960s and '70s by handing out tiny crystals of urea for his students to taste. These crystals instantly make the tongue feel as if it were shriveling up. Then comes a cold sensation and a taste so bitter that no one who has tried it can forget (we know!).

This cold, shriveling sensation is a clue to why urine is a therapeutic agent. The urea creates very high osmotic pressure, literally sucking the water out of the cells of the tongue. As with honey and sugars, the high osmotic pressure created by urea has a debriding effect on open wounds; that, in fact, is one of its most common uses in pharmaceutical preparations today. Urea is found in a wide range of products formulated for treating inflammation of the cervix, postpartum cervical tears, and wounds caused by cauterization and cryosurgery and for debriding skin ulcerations, burns, and postoperative wounds. As the base of one cream, it facilitates the absorption of the hydrocortisone. It is an ingredient in a liquid used to soften and remove ear wax.

The water-sucking action of osmotic pressure can also kill microorganisms. Thus urea, like honey and sugar, acts as an antiseptic and has been used either by itself or in salves and ointments to treat human infections at least since the 1930s in the United States. In fact, when maggots were reintroduced to medical practice in the 1930s, at least one physician objected on the grounds that he believed urea to be a superior debriding and antiseptic agent. Urea is still used as an antibacterial and antifungal agent by some physicians in the United States, Britain, and Russia. Veterinarians use urea ointments to treat infected wounds in animals.

Urea may have specific antiviral effects. One of its most recent uses is as a component of Herpigon, a treatment for herpes simplex infections. According to several scientific studies, this combination of zinc, tannic acid, and urea effectively eliminated all symptoms of genital herpes over a several-year period and lowered the viral infection below detectable levels. These observations suggest that Heath's use of amoroli to fight viral and fungal infections may not be totally unjustified.

Not only do the chemical components of urine fight infection and inflammation, they may also have important sedative effects, for at least two of them help induce sleep. One is melatonin, one of the "hottest" natural hormones to hit the shelves of natural food stores and naturopathic pharmacies in decades. Neurobiologists have long associated melatonin with sleep regulation, and its ingestion has proven tranquilizing effects. Drinking morning urine, which contains the highest levels of melatonin, is likely to significantly raise melatonin levels in the body during the day, creating much the same results as are touted by those who sell melatonin over the counter.

The other component of urine that may have similar tranquilizing consequences is a compound first isolated from hundreds of gallons of urine by Harvard researchers Manfred Karnovsky and J. R. Pappenheimer. Initially called "sleep factor," it was subsequently identified by them as muramyl dipeptide, a breakdown product of bacterial cell walls probably produced by the normal flora that reside in the gut as well as by severe bacterial infections. This bacterial peptide actually mimics many of the effects of serotonin, the metabolic precursor for melatonin. Apparently the immune and nervous systems have evolved to respond to bacteria and serotonin in very similar ways. The common response is advantageous in that the immune system is activated against injury or disease and at the same time one becomes sleepy (thereby conserving energy). Thus when Heath claimed that amoroli ameliorated his symptoms and allowed him to sleep better, and Madame de Sévigné drank her concentrated urine concoction to calm her nerves, their observations may have been more than just wishful thinking.

Urine has a variety of other effects that both folk and formal medicine have utilized. Its diuretic properties have long been known, which may explain its use by European physicians a few centuries ago as a therapy for gout. Since gout is caused by an excess of uric acid often combined with insufficient intake of water, it is quite possible that urine ingestion benefited patients by increasing urinary excretion and thus elimination of the excess uric acid, a goal of modern treatments as well.

Urine often contains reasonable quantities of hormones, too, especially the urine of pregnant animals or women, and these have wide-ranging effects on the body. Some Hindu texts specify using urine from prepubescent children, perhaps to avoid these compounds. The Chinese, on the other hand, found ways to take advantage of the hormone compounds in urine. According to Joseph Needham and Lu Gwei-Djen, two biochemists at Cambridge University, many of the fractionation, or distillation, procedures using urine worked out by Chinese chemists from the sixteenth century on probably would have resulted in highly concentrated and reasonably pure steroid mixtures. The steroid hormones include estrogens, progesterone, and testosterone, all of which help to control the processes of sexual maturation, ovulation, and pregnancy. Thus, the traditional prescription of these particular concentrates in China to treat menstrual irregularities, pregnancy problems, and sexual dysfunction was probably justified. A related use is found in Zimbabwe, where the urine of baboons and rock rabbits is sometimes ingested in beer as an aphrodisiac.

Western medicine makes use of hormones from urine in similar ways. The modern pharmaceutical industry still isolates and purifies estrogens and progesterone from pregnant mares' urine for human and veterinary use. Premarin, for example, is a mixture of estrogens produced by Wyeth-Ayerst for the treatment of abnormal uterine bleeding and is prepared from mares' urine and other "natural sources." These additional sources can include human beings. During the 1960s Serono Laboratories used the urine of postmenopausal nuns in Italy to prepare Pergonal, which consists of equal amounts of follicle-stimulating hormone and luteinizing hormone. The mixture is used to treat certain types of infertility. Injected into women, it stimulates ovulation; in men, it stimulates sperm production. Serono relied on the urine of postmenopausal women to ensure the right mix of hormones. The company chose nuns to significantly reduce the risk that the urine might be contaminated with sexually transmitted diseases, some of which are notoriously difficult to eliminate completely from human preparations.

Urine also contains trace amounts of many other pharmaceutically active compounds that are being developed for therapeutic purposes. At least one of these was isolated by researchers who paid attention to urine's historical uses: urokinase was discovered as a result of the age-old observation that urine has the ability to help break down blood clots and scabs. During the nineteenth century several investigators demonstrated that some component of urine could digest proteins and, in particular, fibrin — the key component of blood clots. The active material was eventually identified as an enzyme after World War II and named urokinase in 1952 by G. W. Sobel and his colleagues. Urokinase is now used medically as a thrombolytic agent, helpful in breaking up blood clots associated with heart disease and strokes.

The modern pharmaceutical uses of urine components thus justify many of the uses of whole urine in the past, from cleansing wounds to promoting sleep. And believe it or not, those "shocking" practices of bathing in urine or using pee diapers for improving one's complexion have been reformulated and re-packaged by the modern cosmetics industry, too. If you have ever used a skin moisturizer or wrinkle remover, there is a reasonable chance that you have put urea on your face. It is a major compo-nent in both prescription and over-the-counter moisturizing creams for the treatment of rough, dry, cracked, and calloused skin and of damaged nail beds. John W. Armstrong, author of a widely known book on urine therapy, has reported that "one of the most exclusive and expensive toilet soaps [produced in the 1930s] was made from the dehydrated salts and fats of the urine of grass-fed cows, and another from the urine of Russian peas-ants." One wonders whether those who used these soaps were aware of their origin — any more than women and men using urea-based creams are today.

The benefits may not stop at your face, either. Armstrong reported that he rubbed himself with his own urine for years, and his skin was as soft and lovely as that of a young girl. And Dr. Scholl's urea-based Smooth Touch Deep Moisturizing Cream keeps feet soft and smooth. Perhaps this use offers a rationale for anecdotal reports that urine is useful for treating blisters. Appar-ently during the Korean War some of the army rangers sometimes had to march till their feet became so painfully blistered they could not go on. According to one army sergeant, they then peed in their helmets, soaked their feet in their urine "to heal and toughen the skin," and marched on. There don't seem to be any medical studies to validate this particular use of urine, but it is theoretically possible that the urine drew out some of the serum from the blisters, relieving the soldiers' pain. Given the antiseptic nature of sterile urine, it might also have benefited blisters that had ruptured, just as urea creams help the healing of surgical wounds.

The use of whole urine in distant times and places has often been dismissed as yet another example of *Dreckapotheke,* a German word for the medical use of revolting, worthless materials. Nothing could be more wrong, for urine is certainly not worthless, medically speaking. Does that mean we should regard it as a medicine today? Does any physician recommend that we drink our own urine or splash it on our skin? To quote Dr. John R. Herman, a urologist and author of one of the few general reviews of urine therapies, "No. Not yet!"

Herman lists no risks associated with drinking urine or using it for other therapeutic purposes, but he is nonetheless reticent to admit any specific benefits. Despite the anecdotal and historical evidence, the scientific data simply aren't there to support unadulterated natural urine as a modern medicine. The true importance of this bodily fluid, like saliva, lies in the pharmacological agents that can be extracted from it — most notably urea, melatonin, muramyl dipeptide, and urokinase. And more will be identified in the future.

For the present we must view the therapeutic use of whole urine as only a last resort: a lifesaver in an emergency when pure or plentiful water is not available; a therapeutic agent when nothing else will work. And if "shocking child-care practices" and the even more shocking practice of modern amoroli still seem revolting, it is only because they open windows onto ancient medicines that in our own day and age have become increasingly sanitized and scientized.

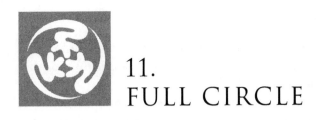

11.
FULL CIRCLE

*With computer technology allowing access to
centuries of available information, it can be shown
that the world's most common operation represents
the essence of prophylactic surgery. The millennia
have endorsed it as a medical/surgical entity of
health enhancement as well as a cultural tool. In
computer lingo, it will be concluded that posthetomy
is indeed "user friendly," while potentially
benefiting society as a whole.*

— Gerald N. Weiss, M.D., and
Elaine B. Weiss, B.S.N., 1994

CONSUMER REPORTS runs a column
called "A Question of Health" that answers
medical questions of every possible sort. One recent letter came
from some distressed parents. "Ten years ago, when our first son
was born," they wrote, "the doctor told us there was no medical
reason to have him circumcised. We believed him. When our second son was born five years ago, we did not have him circumcised
either. Now even Ann Landers advises that circumcision protects
against penile cancer. Did we make a mistake?"

Gary R. Cohan, a physician who writes a regular medical
column for the magazine *The Advocate,* recently received a similar
letter from a gay man also concerned about circumcision: "Since I
was a teenager, doctors have told me to get circumcised 'for health
reasons.' I've resisted them because most guys I sleep with are

really into men who are uncut. Now I hear that having a foreskin puts me at increased risk for contracting HIV. Is this just another safe-sex scare tactic?"

To circumcise or not to circumcise, that is the question. The answer does not come easily, either to parents considering the procedure for their sons or to adults considering the procedure for themselves. At issue may be diverse appraisals of religion, male beauty, physical mutilation, fear of pain, and family tradition. Controversy has arisen throughout history over these issues, reaching a recent peak in the past few decades. Particularly confusing for laymen is that physicians, who call the procedure posthetomy, do not seem to be sure that it provides health benefits.

The problem is exacerbated by ignorance. Despite the fact that circumcision is the most common type of surgery performed in the United States, many people here and in Europe do not know what it entails, and some do not recognize the results. One man recently asked his mother's advice about whether to have his newborn son circumcised, since he, himself, had never been. He was shocked when his mother told him he most certainly had!

Actually, it's pretty easy to tell. Circumcision is a surgical procedure in which the foreskin, or prepuce, is removed. The foreskin is a cylindrical tube of skin that normally covers the dark pink or purplish head of the penis, which flares out at its base and is called the glans. If some skin has to be retracted in order to see the glans, then the foreskin is still intact; circumcised men have nothing to retract. Their glans is always visible. There is a certain absurdity in the fact that the presence or absence of such a small bit of skin should be the focus of so much attention.

The foreskin saga actually begins in prehistory. The earliest evidence of circumcision comes from Egyptian mummies more than 6000 years old. Paintings in Egyptian tombs dating to about 3000 years B.C. illustrate the procedure, as do Pre-Columbian Aztec artifacts. The fact that Egyptians, Jews, and Aztecs performed the surgery using stone knives even into recorded history suggests that the procedure originated in the Stone Age. And a cave painting from some 10,000 to 15,000 years ago has even been interpreted as showing a circumcised male.

Circumcision has had many purposes. Egyptian priests were marking their vocation with circumcision by the time of the Greeks. Jews and Muslims have made the surgery a religious ritual to satisfy their covenant with God or Allah. And for many African, American, and South Pacific tribes, circumcision is a rite of passage in becoming a full-fledged warrior. The earliest written records, however, unanimously suggest that circumcision originated as a hygienic measure. In Greece in the fourth century B.C., Herodotus wrote that the Egyptians "practice circumcision for the sake of cleanliness, considering it better to be clean than comely." (Herodotus's comment betrays the Greek belief that only an unmarred body could be truly beautiful.) Philo Judaeus, another Greek writer, who lived from about 20 B.C. to A.D. 54, was more specific in his book *On Circumcision*. The practice prevented "an almost incurable malady of the prepuce called anthrax or carbuncle, so named from the slow fire which it sets up and to which those who retain the foreskin are more susceptible. . . . It promotes cleanliness of the whole body." Philo even asserted that it increased fertility!

It is worth noting that the matter of penile cleanliness was not — and still is not — something to be taken for granted. The foreskin contains a number of glands on its inside surface that produce a cheeselike substance called smegma. If the foreskin is not cleaned well and regularly, smegma builds up within it, producing a penetrating odor and leading frequently to balanitis, an inflammation of the glans. A complication called phimosis, a narrowing of the opening in the foreskin through which the glans protrudes, can also occur if the foreskin becomes inflamed and swells. Phimosis can cause extremely painful urination and make an erection difficult or impossible.

The connection between cleanliness and healthiness was clearly made in ancient times. Philo explicitly addressed it in his book *Questions and Solutions in Genesis*, where he noted that "it is

135

more difficult and formidable to cure an affliction of the genitals on which a covering skin grows, but this does not happen to one who is circumcised." Many modern urologists have commented similarly on the difficulties that some uncircumcised patients have in maintaining penile hygiene. "As a urologist who sees boys and men at all ages," one of them has written, "I can say that the circumcised penis is clean and the uncircumcised one, all too often is not." Mothers have also made the same observation. One survey found that 40 percent of mothers with an uncircumcised son would circumcise any subsequent sons simply for hygienic reasons.

The distribution of the practice among various peoples of the world provides further clues suggesting its hygienic origins. Philo noticed that while very few peoples in northern countries practiced circumcision, "not only Jews, but also Egyptians, Arabs, and Ethiopians and nearly all those who inhabit the southern regions near the torrid zone, are circumcised." Modern statistics seem to bear out this ancient observation. At present it is estimated that 18 to 20 percent of the world's male population is circumcised. Very few Europeans, Asians, or South Americans are, and the operation is much rarer in southern African nations than in equatorial ones. The majority of those who are circumcised (with the exception of people living in the United States) are Muslims, Jews, northern and equatorial Africans (especially in coastal regions), Australian aborigines, descendants of the ancient Mayans and Aztecs, as well as some American Indians, and the inhabitants of Borneo, Fiji, and Samoa. The vast majority of these peoples inhabit or originally inhabited desert or jungle regions.

Personal hygiene can be particularly difficult in these regions for a number of reasons. In desert areas, where sand gets into everything, grit under the foreskin is no laughing matter. Intense heat causes sweating, which encourages various infections and rashes. Moreover, water for bathing may be scarce or nonexistent, so making it difficult to properly clean the foreskin. Even today balanitis and phimosis are much more common in desert countries than anywhere else in the world save jungle regions. In the tropics the problem is too much moisture rather than too little. In humid conditions fungal, yeast, amoebal, and protozoal infections are extremely common. These parasites and pathogens like nothing better than warm, wet crevices and folds of skin.

The risk of foreskin-related infections is, in fact, the primary reason that circumcision is much more common in the United States than the rest of the Western world. During World War II medical officials of the U.S. armed forces noted that fungal and parasitic infections of the prepuce were so frequent in soldiers serving in the South Pacific that circumcision eventually became mandatory for those shipped to this theater. The practice was also promoted during the Korean and Vietnam wars. As a result millions of American men who would not otherwise have been circumcised were. Back in civilian life, many men had their sons circumcised too, either because they liked the result or because they felt it was important for their boys to resemble them in this intimate way. Physicians, many of whom had served in the military, wholeheartedly endorsed the practice, and neonatal circumcision rates reached about 75 percent between 1950 and 1980. In Canada and Australia, for similar reasons, close to half of all newborn males were circumcised by the 1970s.

Certain technological innovations contributed to such mass circumcision. For most of medical history, Western physicians had actually been wary of cutting away penile foreskin except when medically necessary. Circumcision was surgery, which always carried danger of uncontrolled bleeding, infection, and a misplaced knife. Through the first few decades of this century, circumcisions had to be performed "freehand," so this last risk was very real. By the late 1930s and early 1940s the invention of the Gomco clamp had revolutionized circumcision significantly by minimizing the possibility of injury. The clamp and associated surgical techniques not only protected the glans from potential harm but also cut off circulation to the prepuce, making the surgery relatively painless and nearly bloodless. Indeed, the Gomco clamp and subsequent inventions such as the Mogen clamp were so effective that after 1950 most physicians began to treat circumcision operations as virtually risk-free and pro forma.

Within two decades, however, some physicians began questioning whether routine male circumcision was a surgical fad, a social ritual with no real justification for use in American medicine. Reviews of the existing medical literature revealed no benefits other than the prevention of phimosis and balanitis, and these two diseases were rare in the United States. In 1971 the American Academy of Pediatrics withdrew its general support for circumcision, leaving it up to individual physicians to decide whether and when the procedure was indicated. By 1975 the tide of opinion had turned. The academy's Ad Hoc Task Force on Circumcision wrote a report that was plainly critical of the practice, concluding in a widely quoted statement that there are "no absolute medical indications for routine circumcision of the newborn." The Canadian Paediatric Society followed suit, and many other studies reached similar conclusions over the next ten years. In 1981 one influential review reckoned that since balanitis and phimosis could be treated as the need arose, neonatal circumcision was unnecessary for anyone. Only two nonmedical reasons were given for performing the operation at birth at the request of parents: religious practice and penile hygiene.

No one seemed to notice that these recommendations to drop routine circumcision lacked foundation in research. The fact was that almost nothing was known about relevant risks and benefits; the recommendations were based on ignorance. Nonetheless, the doubts of the medical profession spread to the general public, spurring a huge revolt against the practice. Benjamin Spock, whose *Baby and Child Care* was the medical bible of millions of families, came out against circumcision in 1976. Jane Brody, best known for her essays on nutrition, wrote against circumcision in an influential essay for the *New York Times* in 1979. Edward Wallerstein, a retired business executive and engineer, published a number of very persuasive books and articles condemning circumcision. Soon a series of anticircumcision advocacy groups began disseminating their views to the public and lobbying both medical groups and legislatures for action. Some of these organizations had wonderful acronyms: the National Organization to Halt the Abuse and Routine Mutilation of Males (NO HARMM); the National Organization of Circumcision Information Resource Centers (NO CIRC); and the International Organization Against Circumcision Trauma (INTACT). Individuals were aided in their skepticism by medical insurers, such as Blue Shield of Pennsylvania and the Prudential Insurance Company, which had found an excuse not to pay for the surgery.

Fortunately, some physicians recognized that medical decisions should be based on firmly established facts, not on lack of information. So in the latter half of the 1980s, medical investigators began new studies bent on a rigorous analysis of the risks and benefits of posthetomy. Many of the results were a surprise to physicians, and even more so to nonmedical critics. Wallerstein, perhaps the most vociferous of the anticircumcision crowd, had laid down in 1983 a list of criteria for judging the routine circumcision of newborns. He stated: "If these reasons — ease of hygiene; prevention of venereal disease; prevention of penile, prostatic and cervical cancer; prevention or cure of premature ejaculation; avoidance of adult circumcision; the need for peer/paternal identification; [and] . . . painless and risk free [surgery] — are valid, circumcision should be performed. If they are not valid, circumcision should not be performed." In 1983 the case for the surgery looked dim according to these criteria. After a dozen years of research, however, every single one of Wallerstein's conditions has been satisfied! All, that is, except one: there is no evidence that circumcision prevents or cures premature ejaculation — that seems to be a problem controlled by the mind rather than the phallus. However, circumcision does affect a host of physical conditions.

Without a doubt the clearest brief for the benefits of circumcision involves its protective effects against penile cancer. In 1971 a study found that Muslims in India, who are usually circumcised before puberty, had significantly lower rates of penile cancer than did Hindus (who do not as a rule remove the foreskin). Similar findings were made a couple of years later by comparing rates of penile cancer in Africans who practiced circumcision with those who did not. In Uganda, for example, where sexually transmitted diseases are rampant and very few men are circumcised, the most common form of malignancy in men is penile cancer, a pattern of disease seen nowhere outside of equatorial Africa. Another study found that Jews and other men who had been circumcised as infants were reported to have almost no penile cancer at all. In fact, as of 1975, only six cases of penile cancer in neonatally circumcised men had ever been reported in the United States. These cases obviously demonstrate that the foreskin is not the *cause* of, but rather creates a risk for, penile cancer.

We now know that most penile cancers occur following infections with human papilloma viruses (the cause of genital warts) and other cancer-associated infectious agents. Countries in which circumcision is uncommon and sexually transmitted diseases (STDs) are prevalent, such as Uganda, Zaire, India, and Bali, have very high rates of penile cancer. Even in the United States, one in six hundred men who are not circumcised at birth will develop penile cancer, amounting to approximately a thousand cases per year. Similar figures hold for Canada and Great Britain. In fact, in Australia, as rates of circumcision dropped after 1970 due to the anticircumcision movement, the rate of penile cancer correspondingly increased. We may assume it will increase similarly in the United States and all other countries where circumcision rates dropped. The risk for penile cancer among circumcised men continues to be close to zero the world over.

The answer to the parents who wrote to *Consumer Reports,* then, is that circumcision is the best way to ensure that your son does not get penile cancer. However, in the United States, at least, chances are he will not get such a cancer anyway, and many physicians have argued that rigorous cleaning of the foreskin eliminates whatever risk may exist. If penile cancer were the only hazard mitigated by circumcision, it would probably not be enough to tip the scales one way or another. But there is evidence that circumcision does much more.

Some researchers think that circumcision may help protect men against the development of prostate cancer. The data are much less convincing than those concerning penile cancer, but since prostate cancer is one of the most common cancers among men in Western nations, anything that potentially will reduce the risk is highly welcome. Several preliminary studies have indicated that circumcision is associated with a lower risk of prostatic cancer for all men regardless of ethnic or racial background or country. Further studies have been recommended to determine whether the observed protection is a causal one.

Of more significance than the impact of circumcision on cancers is the fact that an intact foreskin contributes to higher rates of infection. Some types of bacteria actually stick to the foreskin much better than they do to other penile tissues. Every study ever performed has found that urinary tract infections are between ten and ninety times more frequent in boys and men who are uncircumcised. For example, in one group of 144 boys under five years old with definitive diagnoses of urinary tract infections, only two had been circumcised.

Circumcision also confers limited protection against acquisition of some types of sexually transmitted diseases, including gonorrhea, syphilis, chancroid (a cause of genital ulcer disease), candidiasis (yeast infection), and human papilloma virus infections. It is important to note, however, that circumcision does not protect against all STDs. Genital herpes (caused by herpes simplex type 2) is just as common in circumcised as uncircumcised men, as are chlamydial infections and nongonococcal urethritis, a disease that mimics some of the symptoms of gonorrhea. Circumcision is not, in other words, a general preventive for all STDs. It is simply an aid to improved hygiene with specific and limited effects.

Recent research carried out by Gerald Weiss at the Arkansas Cancer Research Center helps to explain the infection risk incurred by uncircumcised men. The inner surface of the foreskin lacks immunological protection, so germs proliferate rapidly on the surface of the uncircumcised glans. But when the foreskin is removed, the glans develops a thicker layer of skin that makes it more resistant to infection. (There is, by the way, no evidence that the circumcised penis is less sensitive sexually than the uncircumcised one, although opponents of circumcision often raise this issue as a scare tactic.)

Whether or not a man is circumcised also affects his partner's risk for sexually transmitted diseases. It should be fairly obvious that if men who are uncircumcised tend to become infected with STDs at higher rates and harbor more infections than men who are circumcised, then their sexual partners will also have higher or lower risks of infection, respectively. Women with uncircumcised sexual partners have higher risks of acquiring papilloma virus infections, syphilis, gonorrhea, chlamydia, and chancroid than women whose partners are circumcised.

In addition, circumcised men also help protect their female sexual partners against cervical cancer. Throughout the world the incidence of penile cancer is almost directly correlated with the incidence of cervical cancer, both of which are linked to the same types of papilloma viruses. In Uganda, for example, with its high rates of penile cancer, the most common malignancy among women is cervical cancer. The relationship also holds true for Balinese men and women, who are mostly Hindus, and for Hindus and Christians in India, where the incidence of both cancers is among the highest in the world. Indian Muslims, in contrast, have almost no risk for either penile or cervical cancer. Countries in which STDs are rare, such as Denmark and Finland, have naturally low rates of penile and cervical cancers, but even in these countries, a woman whose partner is circumcised derives additional protection against cervical cancer.

It is important to be circumspect in the interpretation of these data. Although cervical cancer is much less prevalent in areas of Africa where circumcision is practiced than where it is not, having a circumcised partner is not a guarantee against cervical cancer. The risk is viral infection, not foreskin. Obviously, the protective effect for a woman of having a circumcised partner lessens rapidly the more sexual partners — and infections — he has and the more sexual partners and infectious exposures she has, regardless of circumcision status.

In addition to demanding medical efficacy, Wallerstein and other concerned critics have insisted that circumcision also be painless, essentially risk-free, and likely to be necessary later in life if not done at birth. These conditions are also met in modern practice. First, the operation can be done painlessly. Although traditionally it has been performed without anesthetic even in adults, more and more physicians are using local anesthesia. Innovations such as the Plastibell device and the KLamp further render the question of pain moot.

Second, the safety of the procedure has been validated. The rate of complications in medical settings is less than one in a thousand, the most common complication being heavy bleeding, followed by infection, both of which are easily controlled. The number of cases of penile disfigurement on record is so small as to be not worth mentioning; the proper use of clamps and other devices makes such accidents well-nigh impossible. The real issue is mortality and here the data are very reassuring. A survey taken in New York City during the 1970s found that more than 500,000 men had undergone posthetomy without one fatality. In fact, between 1954 and 1990 only six deaths due to circumcision complications occurred in the United States, and some of these were not performed in medical settings. By contrast, in these thirty-six years between 225 and 317 men died of penile cancer *each year,* all but a handful of them either circumcised as adults or never circumcised. In Great Britain during the same time period, no deaths were reported from circumcision, while thousands of men died of penile cancer, again all but a handful of whom were uncircumcised. Rates of death related to infections associated with lack of circumcision have not, apparently, been compiled.

Third, it is reasonably likely that infant boys who are not circumcised will have to be when they grow up. Rates of adult circumcision for medical reasons range from less than 1 percent in Finland, where circumcisions are rarely performed for any reason, to between 5 and 10 percent of uncircumcised men in Canada. These will include in the future more and more elderly men who require care by others when their mental and physical health deteriorates. A survey of people who provide daily hygienic care for elderly patients almost unanimously agreed that circumcised men were much easier to keep clean than uncircumcised men and that circumcised men in their care developed fewer penile infections.

In short, circumcision confers many medical benefits, improves hygiene, and can be done painlessly and safely; if it is not done, a significant number of men will have to have it done later in life. The case is clear-cut. However, the Canadian Paediatric Society and other medical organizations have not yet altered their position against general neonatal circumcision for a different reason — economics. Several studies have been made of the costs of universal circumcision versus noncircumcision. These studies estimate that the expenditure for routine circumcision is between $100 and $165 per person in Western industrialized nations. The total mean lifetime cost of medical problems associated with lack of circumcision in these same nations is estimated to be about $140, considering an average work-time loss of fourteen hours and an average reduction of life expectancy of less than a month. Since the social benefits do not clearly outweigh the costs in these studies, the Canadian committee has concluded that it is unjustifiable to mandate circumcision as a routine medical procedure.

There are two limitations inherent in these analyses. First, they do not apply to Third World nations, where the incidence of cancers and infections associated with lack of circumcision is often hundreds of times higher than in developed nations. Thus physicians in Africa, India, China, and other parts of Asia have all argued that neonatal circumcision is without doubt the most cost-effective way to prevent many diseases of both men and women. Second, these cost-benefit studies are based on mathematical models that are only as useful as they are complete. The studies upon which the Canadians have relied ignore two additional benefits: the effect of circumcision on the incidence of AIDS and on female sterility, both of which carry extremely high social prices.

A most timely observation is that circumcised men have been found to contract human immunodeficiency virus (HIV) infections at significantly lower rates than similarly exposed uncircumcised men. The protective effect of circumcision has been observed repeatedly in African studies, where 95 percent of the risk for HIV-1 infection can be accounted for by a combination of intact foreskin and genital ulcer diseases such as chancroid and syphilis. Notably, African men who had undergone partial circumcision still had an increased risk of HIV infection compared with men who had been totally circumcised. Men with intact foreskins were also found to be at higher risk for HIV in studies undertaken in the United States and Europe.

By 1994, in fact, thirty studies had been conducted on the possible protective effect of circumcision against HIV. Four of these studies found no protective effect, whereas twenty-two found a strong protective effect, in which the risk of becoming HIV-positive was two to eight times lower among circumcised men. Once again, there is no evidence that the foreskin itself is the risk, but rather that STDs causing ulceration are more common in uncircumcised men, making them more susceptible to HIV. Men with foreskins who maintain a high level of personal hygiene therefore probably have no more risk than circumcised men. The problem is that such care is not exercised universally. So the answer to the gay man who wrote to Dr. Cohan is that circumcision may indeed lower his risks of contracting AIDS, not to mention his risk of contracting syphilis, gonorrhea, and other STDs that raise the odds of contracting HIV. It isn't just health-nut hype or some new way to harass homosexuals. The data are real and they make sense.

The AIDS data alter the economics of circumcision significantly. The average cost of treating an AIDS patient is estimated to be about $200,000, most of which comes from government sources — the public coffers. Over the last decade, about 25,000 men have died each year of AIDS in the United States, representing an annual cost of some $5 billion in health-care expenses. If we divide this figure by 125 million, the approximate number of males in the country, the *yearly* cost per male of this epidemic is about $40. The cost per capita may be even higher in tropical countries in Africa and Asia, where the AIDS epidemic seems more virulent and widespread. If circumcision lowered the risk of infection by half, the lives saved would be considerable and the medical resources that could be refocused on other diseases very large indeed. In consequence, a number of public health authorities both in the United States and in Africa have suggested that widespread circumcision may be the best weapon we have at present against the spread of AIDS.

The reduction of female sterility is another benefit that has been left out of cost-benefit analyses of circumcision. As already noted, female partners of uncircumcised men are at greater risk for acquiring a number of STDs. This has unfortunate ramifications, since STD-induced scarring of the fallopian tubes is the single most important cause of sterility in the world. Indeed, it is estimated that as many as one half of women in the equatorial regions of Africa — the same areas hardest hit by AIDS — are sterile due to untreated STDs. Equally stunning are estimates that more than 20 percent of women in their twenties in the United States are sterile. Untreated STDs are again a major culprit. It is an unfortunate "honor" that Americans lead the industrial world in rates of STDs and sterility alike. Sexual practices have their prices. In this case, the price of in vitro fertilization and other high-tech methods to help infertile women conceive runs to approximately $12,000 per patient per attempt to conceive. Success rates are so low that many women spend close to $100,000 attempting to become pregnant, and very few succeed. It does not take much math to realize that with an epidemic of infertility affecting literally millions of women, any practice that reduces this problem also reduces subsequent health-care costs very substantially — not to mention human misery. Routine neonatal circumcision, while no cure, is certainly a tool that could be used to lower infertility and its skyrocketing social costs.

146

Taken in sum, then, the evidence that neonatal circumcision is medically beneficial is, as Edgar J. Schoen, chairman of the Task Force on Circumcision for the American Academy of Pediatrics, has said, "overwhelming." Whether it should be a routine neonatal procedure or not is another issue, one that should be left to each parent to decide in light of the medical evidence and their own religious, social, and personal convictions. It is not our purpose to convince readers to adopt this or any other medical procedure described in this book.

Rather, our point is that the ancient innovators who invented circumcision were not simply hacking off a piece of skin to appease some god or mark the clan. There were real medical benefits to this cultural practice, some of which our ancestors may have recognized, such as curing or preventing infections, and some of which we are just beginning to recognize today. Moreover, the pioneers of circumcision may have had profound impact on the health and well-being of their cultures, especially in regions where penile infections were common. Men who were circumcised, particularly at a very early age, would have had fewer infections and would have been healthier than uncircumcised men, as a statistical aggregate, and they would have had a slightly greater life expectancy. Moreover, they would have transmitted fewer infections to their women, who, in turn, would have had a significantly lower rate of disease-induced infertility and a lower chance of passing a sexually transmitted disease to their newborns. The cultures that practiced circumcision did not have to understand these consequences in order to benefit from them. They simply outsurvived and outreproduced their neighbors and so took over their regions of the world — something that Philo noted 2000 years ago.

The odd thing about culture and biology, however, is that having married, they can also become divorced. Once people who practiced circumcision migrated to regions in which personal hygiene was easier to perform, and once technological advances made sanitation so much easier to achieve, the biological benefits of circumcision largely (though not completely, as we now know) disappeared. Balanitis and phimosis are not common problems in modern industrialized nations where running water and access to soap are taken for granted. Cultural and religious tradition, however, clearly kept the practice alive in the past and even in our own century. Looking like every other male in one's tribe, or looking just like one's dad, has been at least as important as the medical benefits frankly unintended or long forgotten.

Unintended or not, however, these medical benefits do exist. And so we have come full circle. Excising the foreskin almost undoubtedly began as a medical measure and, thousands of years later, has finally been medically vindicated. How and when we use this ancient medical tool is now up to us.

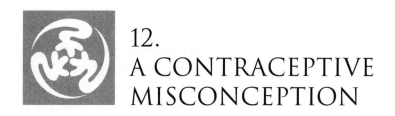

12.
A CONTRACEPTIVE
MISCONCEPTION

It is not inconceivable that a thorough inquiry by medical science into the effectiveness of many recipes commonly thought by anthropologists and others to be magical may teach us much about modern contraception.

— Norman Himes, Ph.D., 1936

NORMAN HIMES was neither a medical man nor a historian. He was a professor of sociology trained at Harvard. So when he set to work on a medical history of contraception in 1930, he naturally turned to the experts. He wrote to forty of the leading medical historians throughout the world, asking them for investigative leads on birth control before the modern era. Contraception was a delicate subject in 1930. Libraries often kept books bearing on the subject uncatalogued and under lock and key. With tact, patience, and persistence, Himes had already managed to ferret out some of them. He was disappointed, however, when only three of his experts, many of whom were practicing or retired doctors, were able to provide him with additional information. Himes discovered that the experts knew almost nothing about contraceptive practices in the past. Was contraception mostly a modern Western phenomenon?

No, for Himes was to learn over the next few years that contraception had been practiced around the world, from primitive to civilized groups, for at least several thousand years. Himes's

Medical History of Contraception, an exhaustive account published in 1936, included chapters on preliterate societies in Africa and the Americas; on the ancient civilizations of Egypt, the Middle East, Greece, and Rome; on the eastern cultures of China, India, and Japan; and on the Islamic and European worlds. The sources were numerous; the methods of contraception various. Women sneezed after intercourse to force out the semen, men denied themselves the moment of ejaculation, couples ritually ate bark and other substances to make themselves sterile. As a sociologist, Himes believed that any human phenomena repeated through time and space were of the utmost interest. But he did not for one moment imagine that all the plugs and potions for which he had found such ample evidence actually worked. What interested him most was that the desire to control conception was universal.

Himes, like the medical experts he contacted, assumed that many of the contraceptive practices he documented belonged to the realm of superstitious, irrational thinking. He believed that effective contraception truly was a modern phenomenon, dependent on the use of inventions such as the rubber diaphragm, the rubber condom, and spermicidal jellies. No society, said Himes, had achieved effective contraceptive measures before the twentieth century. Thus began one of the most persuasive and misleading medical myths of modern times, for most of Himes's conclusions were repeated until very recently by doctors and scholars alike. We know now, however, that the contraceptive myth was misconceived. Many ancient techniques, though far from 100 percent effective, were capable of lowering the probability of pregnancy.

It has long been believed that the only population control practices worthy of the name in the distant past were infanticide and sterile forms of intercourse. Scholars who have studied the infanticidal tendencies of other animal species speculate that infanticide has been deeply rooted in human behavior since the dawn of time. We know for certain that infanticide has been practiced around the world, from tribal peoples in Madagascar and New Guinea to the nineteenth-century Japanese. Infanticide has also had a place in European culture; there is no doubt, for instance, that some unwanted infants were deliberately exposed or smothered in ancient Greece as well as in eighteenth-century France. Evidence that infanticide was a common form of population control is, however, largely anecdotal. It may have been only a last resort practiced after the prohibition or failure of contraceptive and abortive measures.

Among these measures, sterile intercourse seems to have been universal. Indeed, being "careful" in one way or another has been a leading contraceptive choice for thousands of years. Coitus interruptus or withdrawal, which involves the ejaculation of sperm outside the vagina following regular intercourse, has been documented among preliterate peoples in Africa and the South Pacific, as well as throughout Europe from the eleventh to the twentieth century. Anal and oral intercourse have been practiced more discreetly but have had a similar pattern of distribution. Indeed, the deliberate practice of "perverse" forms of sterile intercourse is implied in many apparently irrational contraceptive talismans, such as this one recorded by an alchemist of the thirteenth century: "If a woman hangs about her neck the finger and anus of a dead fetus she will not conceive while they are there." The talisman may have been a reminder for her and her partner that there are other ways to have sex. Similarly, among Amerindians and aboriginal Australians, males have diverted their sexual urges from women to prepubescent, and thus infertile, girls. And in other societies, such as that of the ancient Greeks, men engaged in homosexual intercourse until marriage and sometimes after.

Despite the ancient lineage and practical efficacy of sterile forms of intercourse, however, these methods have never represented the sum total of human contraception. Indeed the most important check upon fertility for thousands of years has undoubtedly been prolonged lactation. Among nutritionally deprived women, frequent suckling on demand can suspend the reproductive cycle. Many peoples, from the ancient Egyptians to the modern !Kung of Africa, have exploited lactation to space their children two to four years apart. However, improved nutrition and early weaning in industrializing societies have made this natural method of contraception virtually unheard-of today — though many scientists enthusiastically encourage a return to prolonged breast-feeding in Third World countries.

Perhaps because of the inexact contraceptive results of breast-feeding, the emotional and moral costs of infanticide, and the male control of coitus interruptus, special forms of female contraception were also developed in the distant past. Ancient Egyptian medical papyri prescribed pessaries, or suppositories, made of crocodile dung, plant fiber, and fermented dough to be placed in the vagina blocking the cervix. The ancient Greeks used tufts of wool, the Hebrews absorbent cotton, the Arabs vegetable pulps, the Japanese and Chinese disks of oiled silk paper, and the Europeans of the 1700s natural sea sponges. Mushroom-shaped stem pessaries made of gold, silver, wood, or ivory were used to support or "plug" the cervix in nineteenth-century Europe and America. In the past hundred years the natives of Central Africa have made pessaries of grass, while poor women of the southern United States have resorted to red clay.

These barriers were often impregnated with other substances. The ancient Egyptians, for example, anointed their pessaries with honey or oily liquids, which acted to seal the mouth of the cervix. A sponge soaked in olive oil was still considered an excellent contraceptive at the turn of the twentieth century in Europe. Other agents such as alum, rock salt, soap, lemon juice, vinegar, and wine also had appropriate spermicidal effect when used with a barrier or alone as a douche immediately following intercourse. The efficacy of douching as a contraceptive procedure has been called into question in our own century, but in 1996 American researchers reported that regular douching, even with plain water, does indeed significantly reduce the incidence of conception.

These female techniques had their male counterparts. According to a medical text that was standard in Europe for centuries, agents such as cedar oil, oil of balsam, and ceruse (a lead compound) were applied to the penis to "corrupt the seed" and

152

prevent pregnancy. There is no evidence yet that such practices were at all effective, and the various forms of penis protectors worn by primitive peoples certainly were not. The first contraceptive male barriers may have been the Chinese oiled silk sheaths dating from the tenth century and the Japanese hard condoms, or helmets, made of shell, horn, or leather. However, some centuries earlier the Romans apparently made condoms out of goat bladders, and the recent discovery of animal-membrane sheaths in the garderobes, or latrines, of English castles suggests their persistent contraceptive use in Europe hundreds of years ago. In the eighteenth century Casanova amused the ladies by inflating his animal-membrane condoms to test for holes, but contraceptive sheaths did not really come into their own until the vulcanization of rubber in the early nineteenth century. It is a little-known fact that Goodyear made not only millions of tires but millions of condoms, too!

Give or take an oiled penis or a dung plug, most of these ancient contraceptives are believable today. After all, we can recognize in them the primitive prototypes for modern cervical caps, diaphragms, and condoms made of latex rubber. We have our own versions of vaginal suppositories and creams and douches. To give him his due, Himes, too, recognized a limited contraceptive value for most of these ancient materials and techniques. Yet he did not find believable one additional form of birth control that has been recorded in medical texts for thousands of years. Recipes for oral contraceptive preparations to be ingested before or after intercourse have been found in the earliest Egyptian papyri, in Greek manuscripts, in European herbals and midwifery manuals, in anthropological records, and in folk traditions around the world. But Himes, writing before the invention of birth control pills, could not accept the contraceptive efficacy of substances taken by mouth.

As far as Himes was concerned, there was no rational contraceptive reason to ingest resins such as myrrh or the sap, seed, or stalk of such plants as artemisia, pennyroyal, Queen Anne's lace, rue, or squirting cucumber. Rather, he believed these potions were

meant to induce sterility "according to some symbolic or sympa-
thetic magic." Himes's conclusions, however, rested upon utter
ignorance of the biochemical activity of many of these plants and
their effect on the female reproductive cycle. He was not alone in
this. The discovery of female sex hormones in plant tissues in the
1930s was skeptically dismissed by many. In the light of scientific
efforts to develop a hormonal contraceptive during the 1950s,
however, the ancient and folk use of herbal preparations previously rejected as superstition began to make rational sense.

Researchers set about examining ancient records more sym-
pathetically. Plants such as barrenwort and birthwort represented
tried and true folk contraceptive aids that scientific medicine
could profitably investigate. Subsequent research revealed, in fact,
that many of these plants did induce menses in laboratory animals
either before or after conception, thus adversely affecting fertility.
In 1992 John Riddle, a historian of science at North Carolina State
University, published an exhaustive study relating this newfound
knowledge of herbal activity to the ancient recipes for birth control that had made their way into European medicine via the
Greeks and the Arabs.

Riddle validated numerous practices, including the use of
pomegranate pulp as an active contraceptive pessary and the ingestion of pennyroyal, Queen Anne's lace, and rue, among many
other substances, as potent birth control agents. Moreover, he
found confirmation of these ancient practices in certain folk cultures today. In the Appalachian Mountains, for instance, and in
rural India some women still eat the seeds of Queen Anne's lace to
ward off pregnancy and to space their children.

In short, historical and scientific studies have substantiated
numerous past contraceptive practices, from breast-feeding to
douching to the ingesting of herbal preparations. The question is,
how did this knowledge — particularly knowledge of oral contraceptives — disappear from learned circles? Why did Himes find it
so difficult to recover and even more difficult to believe? Why did
Riddle have to dig through hundreds of obscure scientific articles
to find out whether any of these practices could have been effec-

tive? Why did he find this knowledge still persisting in isolated, backward places? Finally, why has this folk medicine as a whole been so largely ignored in recent times?

The answer lies in the cultural control of knowledge, and while contraception presents a special case, it illuminates, too, a much more general process. In ancient times birth control was largely the province of a female culture of midwives versed in the special medical concerns of women. The educated men who wrote medical texts in ancient Egypt and Greece learned about contraception from intelligent observation of female folk practices. As long as the ties between folk practice and lettered medicine remained strong, contraceptive knowledge was transmitted by both the spoken and the written word. This was, in fact, the case in the ancient and early medieval world. By the fourteenth century in Europe, however, social and institutional forces began to marginalize midwives and denigrate their ancient birth control knowledge.

Sponsored by the newly emerging universities, medical training slowly shifted from apprenticeship to pedagogy and, just as importantly, excluded women. The female practitioners who attended women in childbirth had no access to new advances in learning or to professional membership in medieval medical guilds. Nor did the male university-trained physicians gain experience in childbirth or birth control. Throughout the medieval period, midwifery remained a female occupation forced to rely on traditional and practical knowledge alone. When, from the sixteenth to the eighteenth centuries, obstetrics developed as a male-dominated profession, it was primarily based on technical and instrumental advances divorced from and considered superior to folk learning and female experience.

During this same period midwives were pressured by religious authorities to relinquish the provision of birth control measures to women. As Christianity emerged from the ancient world, the attitude of the Roman Catholic Church toward birth control had been one of ambiguous acceptance. Early church officials tolerated, even disseminated, traditional contraceptive and abortifacient techniques. By the early Middle Ages, however, church doctrine turned to the control of sexual behavior and against both contraception and abortion, insomuch as they promoted pleasure unassociated with procreative purpose and violated religious notions of ensoulment preceding birth. The church, which by the twelfth century dominated most of Western Europe, tried to repress the transmission of birth control knowledge and influenced secular authorities to make similar efforts.

In town and parish, neighborhood women tending each other in childbirth became subject to the authority of municipal and religious officials, who were suspicious of their practical lore. Church and state required midwives to reveal illegitimate pregnancies and to baptize the stillborn but also to forswear contraception, abortion, and infanticide. Despite these regulations, however, evidence exists that midwives continued to deal in folk methods of birth control. Indeed, strictures against these practices were reiterated for the next 700 years, thus indicating an ongoing battle between midwives and governing officials. Over time the religious authorities won out, successfully tainting the ancient practices as immoral and criminal. Centuries of Christian hostility finally culminated in the wholesale conversion of European governments to secular opposition to birth control.

In England, for example, the Ellenborough Act of 1803 made it a hanging crime to procure or perform an abortion by "any deadly poison, or other noxious and destructive substance or thing" once a woman was "quick with child." This act was significant, both for its affirmation of quickening as a turning point in pregnancy and for its prohibition of abortifacient poisons. For thousands of years popular understanding had confirmed pregnancy and the living status of the unborn by the first felt movements of the fetus at around the fourth or fifth month of gestation. The church accepted this notion through the end of the sixteenth century, only later declaring that life began at the moment of conception. Secular law did not necessarily follow. Thus in 1803 abortion after quickening became a capital offense in

England, but abortion before quickening was considered a lesser crime, punishable only by transportation abroad.

Since Greek and Roman times the uncertain and personal nature of "quickening" had allowed women a flexible period of time within which they might freely exercise abortifacient techniques without sure knowledge of their pregnancy. Traditionally these techniques included the use of emmenagogues or "menstrual regulators," preparations that induced the flow of menses and, if conception had taken place, caused miscarriage. It is precisely these abortifacient drugs that the Ellenborough Act singled out for their "poisonous" nature and condemned. Even in the United States, where physician-induced abortions were tolerated somewhat longer, medical opinion vociferously opposed oral abortifacients as unsafe, even fatal, for pregnant women. Many of these drugs were used in different doses to regulate menstruation and to bring on abortion; some were used for contraception as well. An attack on their use after quickening involved a simultaneous attack on their use before quickening and even before intercourse.

In fact, in both England and the United States the proscription of abortion was closely tied to the repression of contraceptive information and the criminalization of contraceptive practice. By the mid-1860s, when American legislation outlawing abortion both before and after quickening had become widespread, legislators in many states made it illegal to publish or sell pamphlets or books containing "recipes or prescriptions for drops, pills, tinctures, or other compounds designed to prevent conception, or tending to produce miscarriage or abortion." The same association of contraception with abortion occurred on a national level. Under the Comstock Act of 1873 it became illegal in the United States to manufacture, advertise, sell, give away, or otherwise trade in obscene materials of all sorts, including contraceptive information and instruments. A similar criminalization of contraception was implemented by a British law in 1857 and a German law in 1900 against obscene advertising.

Laws, of course, are usually passed in response to social practice. One need not ban what no one does. Throughout the nineteenth century, in fact, sponges, condoms, douches, diaphragms, and other contraceptive implements, like the soluble pessary referred to as "Preventive Mucilage," were euphemistically advertised and obviously sold. Birthrates declined steadily over the century throughout Europe and North America, suggesting that traditional forms of contraception, whether biological or behavioral, homemade or manufactured, were both effective and widely practiced. Family size fell, on average, from five or six children in the early 1800s to two or three over the next hundred years. People were using contraception and plenty of it.

Nevertheless, official government prosecution in the nineteenth century eventually drove public and professional knowledge of contraceptive and abortifacient drugs out of existence. Consider a scandalous trial that took place in England in 1871: the Crown accused a man named Wallis of administering a "noxious substance" to his paramour, causing her to miscarry a six-month fetus. The noxious substance turned out to be an herbal infusion of pennyroyal leaves and two doses of Griffith's Mixture, a readily available patent medicine containing iron and myrrh, a resin used since ancient times as an antifertility drug. The court, however, could not decide just how noxious these oral preparations really were. The prosecution's medical experts testified that both pennyroyal and Griffith's Mixture were potent emmenagogues "sufficient to procure abortion." The defense supplied expert testimony to the contrary. Opinion, even medical opinion, could not establish an abortifacient effect for either the tea or the mixture, although "ignorant women," it was believed, may have used both for that purpose. The court eventually threw up its hands and declared the miscarriage due to the woman's daily horseback rides.

The Crown v. Wallis serves as a kind of benchmark in the history of birth control knowledge. Several decades before the case medical experts uniformly acknowledged pennyroyal to be a menstrual regulator and abortifacient in keeping with the plant's folk use. Several decades after the case, however, doctors uniformly dismissed pennyroyal's effects out of hand. By 1905 a medical jurisprudence textbook belittled the herbal preparation as popular superstition, "never used at the present day by medical men. It [pennyroyal] has neither emmenagogue nor ecbolic [abortive] properties." No wonder, then, that in the 1930s Himes and his medical experts wrote off such preparations without a thought!

The contraceptive and abortifacient properties of other substances were similarly "forgotten" over these critical decades, lost in a flood of unregulated emmenagogues ranging from mild laxatives to systemic toxins. An American doctor named Ely Van de Warker studied twelve of these patent medicines in the 1870s. Only two contained ingredients — oil of tansy, oil of savin (a species of juniper), and black hellebore — that had been used traditionally to promote menstrual flow and miscarriage. Physicians indiscriminately lumped these with other patent medicines, labeling them all as dangerous poisons. Their use was proscribed by licensed doctors.

This repression of medical knowledge was exacerbated by the fact that physicians also lobbied for governmental prohibition of birth control practice by unlicensed practitioners. Abortionists, like the infamous Madame Restell in New York, irregular healers, and anonymous midwives were driven out of business. Physicians in Michigan complained in 1874 that "almost every neighborhood or small village has its old woman, of one sex or the other, who is known for her ability and willingness" to provide birth control. Within decades these folk practitioners had been forced out of practice or out of sight. So complete was their denigration that by the turn of the twentieth century, when college-trained midwives became intent on gaining professional prestige, they had to strive long and hard to dissociate themselves from their disenfranchised predecessors.

Ironically, even the early-twentieth-century birth control movement had a major hand in the marginalization and loss of traditional contraceptive techniques. Margaret Sanger, the American activist responsible for the term "birth control," began her campaign as a supporter of traditional formulations. She provided recipes in a 1914 pamphlet for simple salt or vinegar douches and cocoa-butter suppositories. Similarly, the British birth control advocate Marie Stopes recommended bath sponges and cotton waste soaked in olive oil, salt butter, soap, or vinegar as good makeshift contraceptives — even a hollow rubber ball cut in half could serve as a pessary in a pinch! As the movement matured, however, Sanger and Stopes condemned these methods along with abstinence, extended nursing, coitus interruptus, and condoms as ineffective and dangerous. They and other birth controllers warned the public away from the traditional contraceptive advice of "quacks" and neighborhood women and urged, instead, the patronage of medical professionals and modern methods.

Sanger and Stopes advised using the newer inventions of, respectively, the diaphragm and the cervical cap. These technologically advanced barriers, they argued, put contraception within female control, since the woman decided whether and when to use the device. This, of course, had been true of the many older barrier techniques, douching, and the ingestion of contraceptives and abortifacients. Sanger and Stopes had another reason for their about-face on traditional methods. In fact, they were making overt bids to legitimize birth control by medicalizing it, placing it solely in the hands of the medical community for the first time in recorded history. Prior to the twentieth century, any woman with knowledge of an appropriate recipe could make up a contraceptive douche or sponge, but the modern diaphragm and cervical cap required professional fitting and proper use in order to be effective. In short, they required medical dispensing and medical supervision. The late nineteenth century saw doctors ignore and forget the age-old wisdom concerning contraception. The early twentieth saw birth controllers turn their backs on it as well.

The early twentieth century was, in fact, at a crossroads in public knowledge of contraception. The patent medicines, herbal preparations, and abortion services that had brought about a tremendous decline in the birthrate in the previous century had been vigorously suppressed by moral and legal restraints. Through the 1910s and '20s, the medical profession in Europe and North America opposed birth control in any form. "Respectable" physicians kept their distance from birth control clinics dispensing diaphragms and caps; most refused to discuss the subject in private consultation; a good many publicly declared that contraception — whether male or female — was physically dangerous, morally reprehensible, and causally related to cancer, vaginitis, mania, and nervous breakdown. At the same time, however, powerful commercial interests promoted the invention and distribution of patentable birth control devices such as the diaphragm and cap and the latex condom. No doubt the standardization of barriers and spermicides, along with guidelines for their use, increased their contraceptive effectiveness but the gain was offset by loss of easy access to these and other contraceptive techniques.

Eventually the moral tide against birth control began to turn. In the early 1930s new understanding of the female reproductive cycle and its infertile periods led to the popularization of the rhythm method of contraception. Though initially the response was mixed, Catholic use of the method was sanctioned by Pope Pius XII in 1951. Meanwhile religious opposition to birth control among Protestants had already begun to wane. Over the next three decades laws banning the dissemination and practice of contraception were dropped from the books in the United States, Great Britain, and elsewhere. As early as 1937, the American Medical Association acknowledged that contraception ought to be taught in medical school, but it was not until the introduction of the contraceptive pill in 1960 that the medical profession fully supported birth control once more.

The doctor-supported forms of birth control were, however, severely limited. Three or more generations of physicians had been trained in ignorance of traditional abortifacient preparations and in suspicion of popular contraceptive practices, including breast-feeding, coitus interruptus, and douching. Technologically improved versions of the condom and vaginal creams, available over the counter, met with cautious approval, but the profession's sights were set on the "scientific" methods of the twentieth century: the diaphragm, the intrauterine device or IUD (a modern adaptation of the stem pessary), and the contraceptive pill. When, in the mid-1970s, an American historian named James Mohr asked his medical colleagues whether the emmenagogues and abortifacient potions of the nineteenth century really might have worked, they unanimously said no. Patent medicines and old wives' tales were just that — patent nonsense! Modern medicine had severed all contact with the historical roots of contraception and with folk cultures around the world.

The repression and loss of knowledge are a serious matter, but let us make one thing perfectly clear. We are not claiming that the traditional contraceptives or patent abortifacients ignored by modern medicine are safe and practical in today's world. In fact, we do not recommend any of the old birth control techniques or contraceptive drugs mentioned in this chapter for self-prescribed use. The ingestion of plant materials can be dangerous. In 1978 three women in the United States fell severely ill and one died after taking pennyroyal oil to induce abortion. The inexact transmission of contraceptive folklore had, in this case, led to a confusion between the overly potent oil and the weaker infusion of leaves.

Moreover, it is our perception that women in the past using traditional methods and oral preparations may have gained contraception at the cost of vaginal infections and other systemic injuries, including permanent sterility. Dung plugs may have introduced pathological bacteria into the vagina. Douching may also have increased the incidence of vaginal infections. Pessaries of grass used by African women sometimes led to compaction of the urinary tract and the bowels. Cervical caps and stem pessaries left in place for long periods of time often caused massive infection. At times oral preparations produced violent illness. All of these side effects posed a threat of death.

Why, then, should we be interested in reconsidering this old contraceptive knowledge? Because hindsight is a gift we can use. In the first place, the true history of contraception tells us a story about ourselves. It is easy to recognize ignorance at a remove of twenty or sixty or a thousand years; it is less easy to recognize it in our own time. Yet consider this. Despite the tremendous ferment of medical discovery in the last twenty years, no truly new contraceptives have been developed since the advent of the pill three and a half decades ago. The only exception to this is RU 486, the "morning-after-pill," which seems to work very much like the menstrual regulators of old. As a postcoital contraceptive, or interceptive, it prevents implantation of a fertilized egg and stimulates menstrual flow. As has been known in some medical circles for over thirty years, the same interceptive effect can be obtained by ingesting a combination of regular contraceptive pills. Only recently has this technique come to public light. Clearly the repression of contraceptive knowledge continues to this day.

The history of contraception also teaches, however, that even in the presence of repressive attitudes, men and women in all times and places have desired and acted to control fertility. And when finally mastered, effective and appropriate contraceptive measures have been favored over infanticide and abortion to curtail family size and population. Yet in spite of the sophistication of doctor-advocated contraception in this century, abortion is still a worldwide phenomenon. About a quarter of all pregnancies are unwanted; 50 million a year are aborted. In the United States alone, around half of some 3.5 million unplanned pregnancies similarly terminate in abortion each year. This represents, for American society at least, a troubling rate of contraceptive failure. But until we develop a range of techniques that meet more fully the needs of all people in this country — and around the world — abortion will remain by default a stopgap method of birth control.

What we need, according to a recent report by the National Academy of Sciences' Institute of Medicine, is not more of the same but more of what is different in contraception. And in the effort to broaden our knowledge of the ways and means of fertility control, much can be learned by assessing ancient techniques for hidden, interesting leads. Medical researchers in Africa, China, India, Korea, and Russia are systematically investigating traditional antifertility agents for possible development as modern contraceptives. Western physicians are adapting old ideas — such as vaginal sponges, postcoital contraception, and sperm suppression — to new techniques.

We are not claiming, of course, that all old knowledge is good or accurate or useful. Some ancient birth control agents, such as the zoapatle plant, discovered in the Americas by sixteenth-century Spaniards, and miroestrol, isolated in the twentieth century from a tree root traditionally ingested by Thai women, have already disappointed modern researchers by failing today's standards of efficacy and safety. But we should also recognize that not all modern knowledge is necessarily better. The U.S. Food and Drug Administration announced in November 1996 that many modern contraceptive foams and gels are much less effective than physicians had thought. As the FDA's Lisa Rarick noted, "It's scary to think there are products out there with failures in the 40 to 50 percent range." These products would no more get FDA approval today than would most folk contraceptives. Modern pharmaceuticals are not, therefore, necessarily better than old wives' recipes. The point is that both may provide valid starting points for the development of new and improved birth control methods, and these methods should be held to the same standards of safety and efficacy regardless of their origins. That is not the case at present. Modern methods already accepted by the medical community, all too often without complete validation, have an unfair advantage over any challengers, old or new, simply because they are in use.

The same forces that have served to repress traditional contraceptive knowledge are at work in many other parts of medicine as well. The attack on patent medicines and midwives drove underground not only contraceptive techniques but a large portion of folk medicines and their practitioners. This can only be regretted. No matter how limited their worldly wisdom, people in other times and places have been as capable as ourselves of rational thought and action, and their experience over hundreds and thousands of years has shaped the evolution of our own medical knowledge. The history of contraception repression therefore becomes a cautionary tale of wide significance.

A great deal of learning lies dormant in old records and in folk practice, waiting to be regained. Norman Himes, for one, understood this. Despite his own cultural biases against ancient and folk medicine, which we have only just begun to shed, he realized that some of the most "irrational" medical practices deserve serious study. The alternative is to lose both the knowledge gained by generations past and the control of it for generations to come. "Apart from learning nature's laws," wrote Himes, "I know of no other way of divining the future except by studying the past."

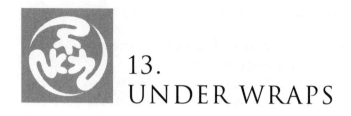

13.
UNDER WRAPS

Sterilized cellophane is an excellent dressing for
clean wounds.

— Edward L. Howes, M.D., 1939

W E WATCHED the dermatologist remove a large mole from our daughter's back. Did the doctor know about honey and some of the other odd treatments for wounds that we were writing about? we asked. "Not much," she said. "But I've got another one for you. The kind of dressing I'm putting over this excision grew out of the World War II battlefield use of cellophane wrappers from cigarette boxes for bandaging wounds." That's right, modern wound coverings and high-tech, breathable plastic bandaging materials impregnated with antiseptics and antibiotics owe their existence to the serendipitous use of cellophane.

Now *this* is a story, we thought! Who would ever link bandages with cigarette wrappers? And yet it had a certain logic. Imagine being a medic in the midst of battle, running out of bandages and having to make use of whatever was available. Cellophane from a cigarette carton? Why not? Almost every GI carried cigarettes. The inside face of the material from an unopened pack or carton might be reasonably sterile, and it was waterproof. Give it a try. Perhaps, we thought, the story might even represent a modern case of battlefield folk medicine leading directly to the latest high-tech treatments.

Moreover, we thought the story might also have something to

166

say about the nature of innovation. Although the epigram "Necessity is the mother of invention" is trite, it is true. Which makes "Who's the father?" all the more pertinent. The answer is, inventions sire more inventions. Inventors make use of available materials, often natural but, increasingly, materials invented by someone else. Invention thus becomes the stuff of further invention. While this paternal image of technological parentage should be as obvious as the maternal image, it gets much less attention. Tracking down both invention and necessity behind the origins of high-tech plastic bandaging might demonstrate, we thought, just how closely the two were wrapped up in the advance of medicine.

To begin with, cellophane was invented in 1898 by C. H. Stearn, a British chemist who figured out how to make clear, thin films from a treated cellulose material called viscose. Discovered six years earlier by three other English chemists, C. F. Cross, E. J. Bevan, and C. Beadle, viscose is essentially a solution of cellulose (the primary ingredient in wood pulp) treated with caustic soda and carbon disulfide. It is a chemical cousin to celluloid, a nitrated cellulose mixture used as the film for many early motion pictures. When spread in an extremely thin layer, cellophane, like celluloid, formed a clear, flexible sheet or film. A Swiss inventor named J. E. Brandenberger designed a machine to produce continuous rolls of the "plastic," and the ability to manufacture useful quantities of the stuff was born. Brandenberger also coined the name cellophane from "cellulose" and "diaphane," the French word for diaphanous, or transparent. Its first use was as a general wrapping material, like paper.

World War I intervened before major production of cellophane could be started, but in 1920 a French company called La Cellophane was founded near Paris, and the product hit the market. The first U.S. cellophane was produced in 1924 under rights obtained from La Cellophane by E. I. du Pont de Nemours & Company at its Buffalo, New York, plant. Du Pont sold it for $2.65 per pound. A few years later the German manufacturer Firma Kalle also began producing the material. The fact that it was waterproof, tough, and clear made it immediately useful. Both permeable and impermeable formulations were quickly invented. By 1940 the cost had plummeted to 33 cents per pound, and cellophane found its way around foods and candies of all kinds and a variety of dry goods. Airplane engines, spark plugs, and even machine guns were soon being wrapped in this miracle material to keep them dry and unaffected by salt air during transport across the oceans to the battlegrounds of Europe and Asia.

Only one major problem plagued the product. During the early years, no sure means of sealing it had been found. In 1929 the Minnesota Mining and Manufacturing Company (3M) began wrapping its masking tape in cellophane, thereby setting the stage for the solution to the sealing problem. One of 3M's employees, Richard G. Drew, looked at the tape, looked at the wrapper, and made the obvious suggestion that an adhesive be placed directly on the cellophane itself. Not only did Drew's invention solve the sealing problem, thus increasing the demand for cellophane, it also led directly to the invention of that still popular product, cellophane ("Scotch") tape. Later on, it was found that cellophane could be sealed by heat, and this method was eventually used on a regular basis for sealing cigarette and other types of packages.

By 1940 cellophane had become a familiar household material. If you unwrapped a loaf of bread, a piece of candy, or a roll of tape, you handled cellophane. If you smoked or handled military materiel, you touched cellophane. It was as much a part of the environment as honey, maggots, mud, or water. It differed only in being new and man-made.

Familiarity bred interest. Just as peoples in the past had liberally experimented with the possibilities of readily available natural resources, so did people begin to experiment with cellophane. Physicians and surgeons were as intrigued as anyone else. Father invention had flexed his muscles and was about to strut his stuff.

The earliest medical use of cellophane we have been able to locate took place in the field hospital directed by Alexis Carrel during World War I. Using cellophane sheets, the French biologist Lecomte du Nouy made daily tracings of wound areas treated with different antiseptic regimens and used the resulting data to attempt a mathematical analysis of healing rates under various conditions. During the next twenty years cellophane was also used to dialyze, or separate out, compounds in various biological materials such as plasma and bacterial cultures, to replace rubber tubing during surgery, and to support tendons and nerves healing after operation.

Other innovations, pioneered by Detroit physician Frank W. Hartman and his son, Frank, Jr., made cellophane even more common in medical settings. In 1940 they noticed by chance that blood delivered intravenously through cellophane tubing slowly desiccated. They made use of this observation to invent cellophane cylinders for the express purpose of dehydrating blood plasma for storage. This invention soon replaced the smaller, inefficient collodion and cellophane bags that had previously been used for such preparations. Cellophane thus became widely used for blood banking. Various modifications made during the war facilitated large-scale preparation of the huge amounts of blood plasma that were needed for the war effort. And, as we will see, the availability of cellophane bags and cylinders in blood units was one of the stimuli leading to cellophane's use as a bandaging material during the war.

Meanwhile a young medical doctor by the name of Dino Donati had pioneered the surgical use of cellophane at the Pathology Institute of the University of Bologna in Italy. Donati, noting certain similarities between cellophane and the dura mater, which forms a diaphanous membrane over the brain, successfully used the plastic as a substitute for the biological membrane during brain surgery. A few years later cellophane was used in Switzerland as a prosthesis for broken eardrums.

The way in which cellophane became a bandaging material is more roundabout. Our dermatologist knew the facts when she said that cigarette wrappers played a prominent role in the history. So did World War II. There is even an element of truth in our imaginary reconstruction of the invention. But the development of cellophane bandaging unrolled with many more twists and turns than we could possibly have imagined.

In the first place, cellophane bandages clearly predated the war. Dr. Helmut Schmidt, a physician working in Munich, first used cellophane as a bandaging material in 1927. How he settled on the plastic is not known, but he obviously recognized that its transparency, porosity, and sterilizability were valuable properties. In addition, he was able to show that using cellophane rather than standard bandages cut down on infections and speeded healing. He and a handful of other German physicians vociferously advocated the new bandages for the next decade, but there is no evidence that they were widely adopted in Germany or that anyone outside the country paid any attention to them whatsoever.

Cellophane bandages were reinvented independently by a British doctor in 1933. A. Vavasour Elder, surgeon commander in the Royal Navy, was in his pantry one day when a container of hot water spilled, badly scalding his shins. He treated himself with several of the standard dressings, but found to his dismay that each of them "caused a state of semi-shock on renewal." This was medicalese for the intense pain he felt whenever he replaced his dressings. The bandaging materials stuck to the healing tissue, tearing it off as they were removed. Looking for alternatives, Elder at some point thought of using "cellophane wrapper from cigarette packets." It was easily sterilized, protected the burn effectively, dulled the pain of the burn itself, rarely needed to be renewed and, when it was replaced, caused virtually no pain since it did not stick to the burn. Over the next five years Elder used cellophane to treat patients with superficial burns, ulcers, and eczema and to cover granulating tissue in open wounds, skin grafts, and surgical stitches.

Unfortunately, Elder did not report his innovation until 1938, after he had retired. Moreover, it appears that his use of cellophane, like Schmidt's, had little impact on the practice of his colleagues. He did note that in tracking down a regular supplier of the material, he had found that the Ohio Chemical and Manufacturing Company of Cleveland was already producing cellophane, both plain and perforated, in rolls designed for surgical use. The company told him, however, that "its use is not generally known in the U.S.A."

Not until a year *after* Elder published did an American, Dr. Edward L. Howes, report his use of cellophane bandaging, which seems to represent yet another independent invention. On January 30, 1939, the journal *Surgery* received from Howes an article entitled "Cellophane As a Wound Dressing." Apparently Howes had noticed a colleague, identified only as Dr. Hazen, covering his patients' bandages with cellophane to keep them from being soiled. This may, in fact, be the "surgical use" for which the Ohio Chemical and Manufacturing Company was producing cellophane. Howes made the logical leap of placing sterilized cellophane directly on the wounds of seventy of his patients, eliminating the standard gauze bandages altogether. He was gratified to find that wound drainage was improved, via the unsealed edges of the cellophane, infection prevented, and healing promoted. Moreover, he could observe the progress of healing without removing the bandaging material. "We believe," he concluded, "it is in every way an economical and satisfactory dressing for the clean wound."

By the time Howes's article appeared in print, the war in Europe had begun. There is no evidence, however, that anyone in a position of authority recognized the importance of Schmidt's, Elder's, or Howes's invention. The only reference to any of these prewar articles that appeared during the next seven years was that of Dr. Edwin A. Nixon of Seattle, who in 1942 proclaimed Howes's use of the plastic one of the "Three C's" of modern surgical healing: "Vitamin C; Cotton sutures; and Cellophane." Nixon's enthusiasm seems to have been unusual. Elder, for example, had noted that patients tended to resist his use of cellophane because it wasn't what they expected a bandage to look like. It is probable that many physicians and surgeons shared this resistance to innovation. Why toy with dressings that already worked — for the most part?

In the meantime, the war introduced Mother Necessity. The need for economical and effective wound dressings quickly became pressing, in some cases desperately so. Still, no one picked up on Schmidt's, Elder's, or Howes's invention, though it was only a matter of time before the advantages of cellophane again became clear, this time under conditions and by people who were less likely to be ignored.

The use of cellophane to treat wounds was independently and almost simultaneously reinvented by physicians in three different parts of the world during the first years of the war. In Nigeria, British wartime economies seriously reduced the availability of bandaging materials supplied to the Colonial Medical Service (CMS). In 1942, Dr. M. Ellis, who worked for the CMS in Lagos, began searching for cheap alternatives to gauze bandages. Recalling Donati's use of cellophane as an artificial membrane during brain surgery, Ellis decided to see if it would act like an artificial skin for wounds and skin ulcers. In the absence of any obvious commercial source, he turned to his local armed forces' canteen, which provided him with "a supply of undamaged wrappings removed with care from packets of cigarettes sold there. We found that these pieces of tissue could be sterilized without damage by boiling in the standard ward sterilizer." He quickly determined that cellophane had five advantages over gauze dressings: "(1) The dressing is non-irritant and simple to apply; (2) the wound can be inspected without uncovering at any time; (3) the amount of discharge [pus] is much reduced — a possible corollary to this is that the smell in the ulcer wards is very much reduced now; (4) a tremendous saving of dressing material; (5) we believe that the rate of healing is increased by the dressing."

Ellis's superiors were so impressed with his results that he obtained permission from the director of medical services in Nigeria to track down a ready source of cellophane. Ellis found that the cigarette wrapping he had been using was marketed under the trade name Rayophane and imported by the British American Tobacco Company, which had a local office. In what has to be one of the oddest partnerships in medical history, the company agreed to provide Ellis, free of cost, the cellophane scrap from their factory for both inpatient and outpatient treatment. No hospital could afford to turn down a deal that good!

A report of Ellis's innovation in the *British Medical Journal* in 1943 came almost immediately to the attention of Major John Farr, M.D., of the Royal Army Medical Corps. Farr at once extended the use of cellophane to burn treatments with great success. Just three days before the Normandy landings of June 6, 1944, he published his work, with a prophetic note that such treatments were amenable to first-aid treatment "anywhere." A "simple measure which could be applied in very forward areas when no medical equipment is available should be considered," he wrote. "In such circumstances the 'cellophane' wrapping of a cigarette package could be applied to the burn for its inner surface is almost certainly sterile; such a dressing would be comfortable and adequate until the patient was able to receive further treatment." Presumably the Royal Army Medical Corps disseminated Farr's ideas among the medics and physicians accompanying the invasion. But, as we shall shortly see, his expedient was already being tried in the field.

The second independent wartime reinvention of cellophane for treating wounds appears to have been made by Captain H. Bloom, also of the Royal Army Medical Corps. Again necessity and accessibility cooperated. Bloom was captured during the North African campaign against the German general Rommel in 1943 and interned as a prisoner of war in Italy. Many of his fellow prisoners were suffering from burns of various types, and Bloom believed that their treatment by the Italian doctors was counterproductive. His reasons were similar to those that had led doctors during and after World War I to reassess the benefits of laudable pus and the closed wound care of plaster casting: "Routine daily dressing of extensive second-degree burns was killing many of our men."

We may presume that sterile facilities did not exist at the POW camp and that sanitation was poor at best. Under such conditions, constantly covering and uncovering an open wound or burn only led to bacterial contamination, infection, and, far too often, death. Experience during World War I had shown that even in sterile conditions constantly unwrapping and rewrapping wounds impaired healing. So to head off this treatment, Bloom devised the ploy of covering the burns with the only reasonably sterile thing available: cellophane obtained from cigarette packages. The results of the sham surprised Bloom, who unexpectedly found the outcome "so gratifying that I became convinced of its value."

Upon repatriation to England in 1945, Bloom gained permission to experiment with burn patients, placing sterilized cellophane obtained from blood transfusion units over second-degree burns treated with powdered antibiotics. Like Farr, he was able to show under controlled conditions that the cellophane helped to prevent infection, eliminated most pain associated with the burns, decreased fluid and protein loss associated with unhealed burn tissue, and increased the rate of healing dramatically. The advantages were similar to those that doctors had seen a generation earlier with the plaster-cast method of immobilizing wounds. Cellophane wrappings hardly ever needed to be changed and, since they were not sealed at the edges, they allowed pus to drain freely out of the wound.

Enter our third reinventor. At the same time Ellis was working in Nigeria and Bloom was experimenting on his fellow POWs in Italy, a Soviet physician, N. L. Chistyakov, improvised the use of cellophane for treating bullet wounds and postoperative lesions in Russia. Although Chistyakov did not work at the front, he took care of evacuated men who had sustained both superficial and deep gunshot wounds needing surgery, and like Bloom and others, he soon realized that ordinary gauze bandages caused more problems than they solved. "Layers of gauze applied directly to a wound," he observed, "may soon become saturated and lose their absorbing capacity. The gauze adheres to the wound surface and causes traumatization during subsequent dressings, the granulating areas become damaged, bleed, and may become infected. The removal of adherent gauze layers causes considerable pain."

174

He soon discovered the advantages of cellophane. One twist on the therapy that he and his colleagues added was to spray the wounds with thrombin, a blood-clotting agent, to lessen bleeding. Another was to replace rubber tubing with cellophane tubes, just as Hartman was doing in Detroit. In addition, Chistyakov saw the benefits of using cellophane for first aid. He specifically recommended that it be used on "fresh gunshot wounds," both for the direct benefits of the material and because such "wound[s] can [then] be examined through the cellophane and watched at the several evacuation points." While we have no direct evidence that cellophane was actually used on the Russian front, it seems likely.

It is worth mentioning one last intrepid innovator at work in the United States in 1942. Drawing on unidentified earlier papers concerning cellophane bandages (presumably those by Howes and Elder), Lieutenant Commander J. W. Kimbrough of the United States Navy Medical Corps also began experimenting with cellophane bandages. His innovation was to make those bandages *self-adhesive*. Taking advantage of the previous work by Richard Drew at 3M, he invented a way of transferring the stickum from cellophane tape to the edges of cellophane sheets. Kimbrough's invention was thus the clearest, most immediate ancestor of modern plastic bandages; but even so the route to our personal medicine cabinets had a long way to unwind.

The results of all of these experiments with cellophane wound dressings were published between 1942 and 1944, and the armed services continued to develop the new bandages throughout the early postwar years. However, medical interest in cellophane bandaging seems to have diminished with the war's end. There were no longer huge numbers of gaping wounds demanding immediate attention, and the new antibiotics took care of most infections. The use of cellophane soon became associated more with surgical *tape* than with bandages. Self-sticking plastic tapes of cellophane or vinyl began to be used more and more frequently to cover surgical sutures. And here once again an unexpected discovery was made. In 1964, a bacteriologist named Richard Houghton began using Scotch tape to seal petri dishes in which he was growing various bacteria. Lo and behold, tape-sealed petri dishes containing *Staphylococcus aureus,* a very common infectious agent in surgical wounds, failed to grow any bacteria. Subsequent studies showed that the bacteriostatic agent was a volatile substance released as a gas from the tape. The oddest part of the story was that this agent, which has apparently never been identified, killed only *Staphylococcus aureus* and no other strain of bacteria tested. So tape on wounds not only protected them generally from infection, it actively fought one of the most common types of infections that surgeons encountered! Perhaps the same had been true of cellophane dressings, too.

The postwar years also saw another major change in bandaging practice. Antibiotics did such a good job of preventing most infections that nurses and physicians trained during that period were usually taught to keep wounds *uncovered* so that they would dry out and form a hard scab. Almost paradoxically, it was argued that keeping a wound covered (and therefore inaccessible to external contamination) and wet would provide a breeding ground for germs, whereas keeping it open (and accessible to germs) and dry was safer. Those who advocated closed wound dressings, such as cellophane or Orr's and Trueta's plaster-cast treatments, fought a losing battle. Only a handful of papers on these topics appeared between 1945 and 1960.

In the meantime new plastics appeared on the medical scene. Vinyl, which had been invented in 1927, found few medical uses until a quick-drying spray form was developed during the 1950s that could be used as a spray-on bandage. Nylon and polystyrenes were introduced in 1938, polyesters and polyethylenes in 1942, epoxies in 1947, and polyurethanes in 1954. Both the polyethylenes (called polythenes in Britain) and polyurethanes could be made into thin, clear sheets similar to cellophane, and once again physicians began to experiment with their bandaging properties. Interest in wet (or occlusive) dressings was reawakened in 1959 by several investigators who compared wound healing under fabric and plastic dressings of various sorts and found that plastic wet dressings were the most effective at preventing infection and stimulating healing. The watershed occurred in 1962 when Dr. George D. Winter, a member of the Department of Biomechanics and Surgical Materials of the Institute of Orthopaedics (University of London) in Middlesex, England, published a paper in *Nature* demonstrating incontrovertibly that covering a wound with polyethylene film was far and away better than the dry approach. Oddly he did not test cellophane and made no reference to it — perhaps because his work was being funded by a manufacturer of polyethylene. In any case the subsequent revolution in wound care took less than fifteen years. By 1979 an editor for the *British Medical Journal* was able to write that traditional forms of wound treatment, such as dry wound care and gauze bandaging, were finally and completely out of favor, universally replaced by modern dressings incorporating "non-adherent film."

Although cellophane continued to be used for some bandaging purposes and for burn care through the 1970s, most practitioners in Western countries moved on to films derived from the new plastics. Some incorporated silicone reinforced with nylon. Polyethylene films were bonded to viscose fibers (the original material from which cellophane is made) for absorbency. Dow Corning, which had been an early supplier of cellophane for bandages, developed a Silastic foam dressing in 1974 called Q7-9100, which was "contour forming, soft, resilient, absorbent, and non-adherent." At the same time Swedish researchers had developed ways not only to wick away excess fluid from wounds but to remove germs as well. Their work led directly to the development of a dextran-based plastic bandage containing antibiotics called Debrisan. Other dextran-based bandaging materials followed quickly, including Opsite, Tegaderm, Biobrane, and many of the wound coverings used today. Cellophane faded away, both as a bandaging material and as a surgical tape, but its progeny have multiplied madly.

For complete coverage of the issue, take a close look at your store-bought bandages sometime. Band-Aids, consisting of nothing more than a gauze pad stuck to cloth tape, were invented during the 1920s by a Johnson and Johnson employee. Now the tape is usually a plastic material, and the gauze pad is a viscose or cellulose product covered by — no, not cellophane but its successor, polyethylene film. Thus, from the battlefields we finally reach the medicine cabinet. Every time we bandage a cut, we make use of a medical therapy that stems directly from the marriage of technological invention and the necessities of war.

That's the sublimity of the mundane. People, like nature, innovate under odd, particular conditions, and the innovations are sometimes copied by society at large. It would be a mistake, however, to consider each instance as entirely unique. There is a general logic to the process, and cellophane dressings help to reveal it as an evolutionary one. A constant supply of inventors provides innovations that compete with one another for survival in the economic and social world. In this instance, between World Wars I and II the economy was revolutionized by thousands of inventions, including plastics such as cellophane. Cellophane survived and flourished. The stuff was (re)produced in such quantities that nearly everyone had access to it and was aware of some of its unique properties. All that was needed was necessity — some problem the nature of which required these properties. Sure enough, World War II came along, and a new ecological niche became available, as evolutionary biologists might say.

And so it happened that on battlefields and in hospital wards, medics and physicians struggled to find novel, faster, better ways to treat horrible wounds and tropical infections. Perhaps they remembered a colleague using cellophane for some reason. Perhaps they held in their hands a cellophane blood or plasma packet. Or perhaps, when they needed a break, they went out to smoke. It was only a matter of time before someone held the problem in their head and the solution in their hand at the same moment. And that moment came independently and repeatedly to physicians and medics the world over. Like a new and better combination of genes, the idea was better suited to the times than anything else. Cellophane was cheap, available, and effective, and it allowed the wound to be monitored without the interference of a dressing change. Nothing else could do all this. In the new field of competition for treatments created by the war, cellophane often won. Then this new hybrid of problem and prior invention multiplied and spread, leading to a new race of plastic bandages.

We tend to forget these first moments of union between Father Invention and Mother Necessity, perhaps because the new-born innovation itself often becomes such a part of our lives that its manifestations become commonplace and unremarkable. Who knew that Band-Aids and high-tech bandages could trace their family history back to the cellophane on a cigarette package on a battlefield in Europe, America, or Africa? Thanks to our dermatologist, their story is no longer under wraps.

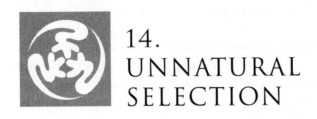

14.
UNNATURAL
SELECTION

WHAT DO CUPPING, artificial leeches, low-pressure barometric chambers, breast pumps, and "pneumatic forceps" for delivering babies have in common? If you answered that they all appeared in a *Connections* essay or TV special by James Burke, you would be close. Actually Burke has never written about these particular inventions, but they have the odd sort of relationship that is his trademark. In this case the common denominator is bloodletting and the connection is evolution. Medicine evolves — literally. And the historical path from bloodletting to suction forceps provides a handy case in point.

The earliest forms of bloodletting involved lancing a vein. With time, various modifications appeared. One of these, dating back millennia, was cupping. In recent centuries the physician heated a glass jar and placed it over scarified skin, usually on the back. As the jar cooled, the air pressure inside dropped and the resulting partial vacuum created a suction that helped draw the blood from broken capillaries in the skin. This sort of "wet" cupping was obviously related to "dry" cupping, in which the partial vacuum merely created welts or bruises on unbroken skin. Practitioners believed that these welts drew the bad humors away from underlying organs, thereby relieving the congestion that was commonly thought to cause disease.

Then leeching came into vogue and largely replaced this and other forms of phlebotomy during the late eighteenth and early nineteenth centuries. But one thing led to another, and by the time leeches grew scarce in the mid-1800s, inventors had already set to work on "artificial leeches." These mechanical devices were often miniature versions of the wet cupping apparatuses of a century before, with the addition of a tiny incising device within the cup itself. So attached were these inventors to their animal inspiration that the incisor frequently mimicked the actual three-pronged bite of a leech.

Meanwhile, another set of inventors realized that the laborious heating of cups could be dispensed with: a better vacuum could be generated by pneumatic pumps. Thus, around the middle of the nineteenth century, bloodletting, mechanical leeching, and pneumatic pumps converged in the creation of pneumatic leeches. These new devices had one major disadvantage, however. Unlike small glass cups, which remained attached to the patient by their own vacuum, the large and heavy pneumatic leeches had to be held on to the patient by an attendant. The next generation of innovators appended small glass syringes capable of reaching into the mouth, anus, and vagina. This represented a real breakthrough, since earlier pneumatic leeches had found these orifices, where real leeches had classically been used, inaccessible.

Put one of these newfangled leeches into the hands of an obstetrician, and the next thing you know he's found another use for the device. The most distressing obstetrical problem has always been how to deliver a child stuck in the birth canal. Physicians have typically used either their fingers or large forceps that vaguely resemble barbecue tongs to grab the infant's head. Between 1848 and 1955 dozens of patent applications were filed by obstetricians around the world who thought they had found a better way: vacuum suction! Modify those uterine leeches and pneumatic pumps, get rid of the incising devices, and voilà, you've got the vacuum "forceps" found in delivery rooms today. As farfetched as it may seem, sucking babies safely into the modern world clearly derives from the long-gone craze for cupping blood.

Take the same devices and apply them to another part of the female anatomy, and yet another set of innovations emerges. Leeches and cupping were used on breasts just as commonly as on any other part of the anatomy, particularly when women developed inflamed nipples during lactation. Almost as soon as each of the artificial leeches described above was invented, someone found a way to modify it to use on breasts, and within a very short time the breast-milk pump was born. Sixty patent applications were filed with the U.S. Patent Office between 1934 and 1975 for such apparatuses, which are of course still used.

The cumbersome pneumatic leeches also changed over time. While many inventors tried to make them smaller and lighter, a Frenchman named Victor-Théodore Junod bucked the trend and made them larger. In fact, he made them large enough to put suction on a whole arm or leg and eventually on the whole body — dry cupping taken to extremities! Whether this sort of vacuum treatment had any useful medicinal effects is highly conjectural, but the technology was certainly related to the subsequent development of low-pressure chambers, which were a mainstay of physiological researchers at the turn of the twentieth century.

Somewhere along the line cupping glasses and artificial leeches diverged a long way from letting blood. Very recently, however, we have seen a return of both the leech and its mechanical mimics for just that purpose. Various forms of reconstructive surgery, such as that following mastectomies, can result in internal venous congestion. Miniature artificial leeches, which are essentially high-tech versions of the old pneumatic ones, can actually be implanted within the reconstructed tissue to drain off stagnant blood and promote circulation. When recovery is complete, the artificial leech can be removed, without all the bother of handling the real thing.

This very brief sketch of the invention trail from phlebotomy cups to vacuum obstetrical extractors, breast-milk pumps, and modern artificial leeches suggests many parallels between medical and biological evolution. One is the unexpected relatedness of medical treatments and apparatuses that are as different in appearance as mammalian whales, humans, and bats. Another is the emergence of viable medical species from practices that have become nearly extinct, a process with remarkable similarities to the way modern reptiles diverged from and outlived the dinosaurs. And yet another is the synergism of unrelated innovations, such as pneumatic pumps and leeching cups, that come together to form new novelties as dependent on one another, as symbiotic, as the algae and fungi that form lichens or the gut bacteria that allow ruminants to digest hay.

In fact, medical evolution, which is cultural, works in essentially the same ways as biological evolution to develop and sustain its particular species. As medical anthropologist Alexander Alland, Jr., has written, an evolutionary process requires variations that are transmissible from generation to generation and some form of nonrandom selection that discriminates between these variations, optimizing the survival of those that best fit their environment. We believe, as does Alland, that medicine is a perfect example of an evolving culture because it has the necessary ingredients — transmissible variations and nonrandom selection. By trial and error human beings have, for thousands of years, created many, many variations in medicinal treatments. By choosing among these variations and passing the more successful ones to their offspring or their apprentices, they have exerted a cultural selection upon the course of medical development.

The histories of many medicinal agents and practices illustrate this evolutionary process. In a common pattern of invention, people somehow discover the healing power of mineral-spring bathing or a medical use for cellophane. They try these things on a wide range of illnesses, injuries, and wounds. A few of the experiments work and some practices are retained. Take, for instance, the evolution of medicinal honey usage, starting in the Stone Age. Wherever honey was available, it was only a matter of time before the sticky sweet substance found its way into the cuts, scrapes, or burns of women and men preparing and eating food. The honey made the wound or burn feel better, so it was tried again. The more perceptive wise women, shamans, and healers may even have noticed that honey kept down infection and speeded healing. After a while the application of honey became a purposeful practice.

Actually, wound healing was only one cell in the complex honeycomb of ancient honey usage. By 1500 B.C. the Egyptians also used honey to purge the body, to bind materials into casts for broken bones, "to drive away bitterness" and pain in the stomach, to alleviate excessive urination and fluid accumulation, to cure headaches, to stimulate hair growth, to beautify the skin, to cure ingrown toenails, to treat insect bites, to treat infected wounds, and to prevent pregnancies. Above all, they already knew thousands of years ago that "a spoonful of sugar makes the medicine go down"! The primary use of honey was to deliver other oral medicaments.

As we noted in Chapter 3, honey was discovered and rediscovered for medicinal purposes by many people in many cultures. These multiple rediscoveries were not always identical. For example, modern rural New Englanders and the Amish people take honey to induce sleep, soothe an upset stomach, and relieve constipation; to treat colic, muscle cramps, and bedwetting; and to alleviate coughs, congestion, and asthma. They also use honey as an antiarthritic agent and a burn treatment. Most of these uses were unknown to the ancient Egyptians, just as some of their uses are unknown to New Englanders and the Amish today. Nevertheless past and present usage overlap in the treatment of burns and stomach pain. Not surprisingly, science has justified one, if not both. Honey is now used in burn therapy in modern Western

184

hospitals. And, if we consider the evidence from eastern European nations, it may have validity in ulcer therapy as well. Over the millennia the truly effective uses have survived in many cultures.

The same process of evolutionary variation and selection can be condensed from centuries to years by modern research methods. Withering's research on foxglove (digitalis) preparations for treating heart disease provides an example. The astute doctor experimented with many varieties of foxglove and many methods of infusion before finding the right therapeutic dose. Then, in addition to treating heart or circulatory complaints, Withering tried the drug for tuberculosis, ovarian cysts, excessive phlegm associated with colds and bronchitis, hydrocephalus (water on the brain), kidney stones, acute renal failure, epilepsy, vomiting, and lead poisoning. Most of these experiments did not work. In the end the valid uses of digitalis could be counted on the digits of one hand.

As crazy as they may seem, however, the *invalid* uses of phlebotomy, leeching, digitalis, or honey cannot be laughed away. Thus far we have emphasized almost exclusively those folk remedies and ancient medicines that have survived the tests of time to become integrated into modern medicine. If we are really to understand how medicine evolves, however, we must also look at how variations in treatments arise and are tested, dismissed, and displaced. Failure, from the evolutionary point of view, is as important as success, for it is only through competition, survival, and extinction that progress in medicine takes place.

In no case is the evolutionary process linear or simple. If we were to plot our examples of medical discovery or invention on an imaginary graph, we would see at the beginning the point where someone makes an observation of possible therapeutic importance. That observation is followed by many more, forming a thick line of corroborating data that lengthens with time. At some point branches diverge from the main trunk as people explore other uses for their remedy or device. Some of these branches become thriving modifications of the original therapy, as exemplified by the development of different types of plastic bandages after cellophane or of different suction devices after the artificial leech. Others fail almost as soon as they bud, as when Withering found that digitalis had no effect on tuberculosis.

The result of this process of innovation over time is a treelike graph — exactly the kind that Charles Darwin used to illustrate his theory of biological evolution by natural selection at work on random genetic variations. In this instance the branches are the medical innovations that survived long enough to make a mark on history. The blank areas between the branches, what artists would call the "negative space" in the picture, are the experiments that did not or could not work or did not work well enough. People died despite treatment, could not abide the treatment, could not get access to it, could not afford it, or could not sanction it. There are many reasons for treatment failure. Eventually, they all lead to the same end: extinction of the therapy.

The important point is that the selection process in the evolution of medicine is exactly analogous to that in nature. Cultural and biological evolution are, in fact, inextricably entwined, for the bottom line in medicine is simple biological survival. Medical therapies that increase the probability that an individual will live to reproduce will give not only the individual but the culture that practices that therapy a biological advantage over cultures that do not. By learning what works as medicine and passing on that knowledge, a group increases its biological fitness.

It would be a mistake, however, to think of this process as simply "eat this, live or die, then go on to the next," cautions Steven King, a vice president at Shaman Pharmaceuticals. The researchers at this company specialize in collecting and testing the medical knowledge of witch doctors and wise women for leads to drugs that may have modern utility. Native healers, King emphasizes, very carefully note which plants and plant parts the animals eat at various times of year or when suffering from specific diseases. These observations help the healers to determine what botanicals may be used safely and what doses to try. Healers often test their concoctions on themselves in order to study the effects of their treatments and decide how to modify them to their needs.

According to the anthropologist and ethnobotanist Paul Cox, the accumulation and transmission of medical knowledge was traditionally not just an individual effort but a social process, and it still continues in the old way in some nonindustrialized societies today. He describes this process as a sort of "historical bioassay" in which knowledge accumulated over centuries of empirical practice was strained through the sieve of "an extensive selection process for safety and efficacy." Whatever worked as medicine was incorporated into general practice and transmitted from generation to generation by means of ritual or schooling.

Sometimes medical knowledge was transmitted overtly, as with the many ancient prescriptions for honey. Sometimes it was implicit. Many rituals apparently divorced from any medical rationale had significant medical — and biological — value. Circumcision was one of these, as were certain nutritional practices, such as the making of beer by early agriculturists or the processing of corn with ash by Amerindians. Nutritional anthropologist Sol Katz of the University of Pennsylvania has argued that the microbial process involved in beer making provides a large boost in mineral and vitamin content, while treating corn with ash releases significant amounts of otherwise unavailable niacin, a vitamin necessary to prevent the wasting disease known as pellagra. Those who prepared their grains in these ways did not need to know the nutritional results in order to benefit through better health and improved survival.

The accumulation and transmission of medical knowledge affect survival positively. There is, in consequence, a sort of "biorationalism" at work in the evolution of medicine, which becomes more and more overt as the criteria for choosing between therapies become increasingly explicit. In the beginning, when there are no treatments for a disease, any practice that is beneficial in even the slightest way will be adopted. Something that relieves the symptoms even if it doesn't treat the causes of the disease is better than nothing at all. Honey may be retained in many preparations, for example, simply because it tastes good. Licking a wound may make it feel better. But once a more beneficial therapy is discovered, the medical environment alters. The competition for social recognition and practice heats up.

Consider an example. At least 2000 years ago, Greek surgeons had learned to relieve the gross water retention of ascites by puncturing or "tapping" the abdominal wall, inserting a hollow reed, and drawing off fluid. The procedure was fraught with complications, ranging from hemorrhage and intestinal lesions to infection and circulatory collapse. In consequence, over the centuries many other, less invasive therapies took a stab at reducing the incapacitating fluid retention. Physicians prescribed purgatives; they tried phlebotomies and leeching; they advised bathing in mineral springs. None of these techniques was demonstrably better than the others, though they did not incur the risks of tapping. When Withering discovered the diuretic effects of digitalis, he tried it on liver disease patients and got much better results.

By the mid-nineteenth century physicians were mixing digitalis and a host of mostly herbal diuretics into special wines, teas, and pills and prescribing them in preference to leeching or bathing for ascites. Some of these treatment modalities — surgical tapping, purgatives, and herbal diuretics — survived well into the twentieth century, when they were finally dealt a near-death blow by the introduction of highly potent mercurial diuretics and their successors. Today any new treatment for ascites — including the recent reevaluation of old treatments such as tapping — must compete, not with phlebotomy, bathing, or digitalis, but with modern drug therapy. Each new generation of treatments raises the standard of competition.

In fact, each surviving innovation in an evolutionary system is itself a new selection criterion that must be bettered by subsequent competitors, thereby ensuring progress. Balneotherapy survives today only in countries that cannot afford modern drugs, and it is being reconsidered in richer countries only for patients who do not respond to them. The emergence of new and more effective treatments has dramatically decreased the viable range of old treatments. Survival of the culturally — that is, medically — fit treatment is exactly analogous to survival of the fittest biological species.

To compete, new treatments must be demonstrably better than the ones we already have. Anything less represents an evolutionary disadvantage. Food and drug agencies in various modern countries have, in fact, formulated guidelines for drug testing and approval in order to prevent such backsliding. In our modern version of biorationalism, a therapy is investigated not by a single shaman but by research teams, and trials are performed on representative populations rather than individuals. The results are no longer transmitted by ritual or by mouth, but by writing, on computer disks, and by professional training. Our standards of efficacy, reproducibility, and safety are enhanced, and progress is that much faster.

So far, so good. Medicine has means of variation, selection, and transmission and therefore satisfies the criteria for being an evolving entity. But there are major differences between cultural evolution and the evolution of species. To begin with, the modes of transmitting adaptive traits are quite different. In biological evolution, individual adaptations are genetically encoded in the individual who survives. The survival and reproduction of the individual carrying that trait is therefore the means of spreading the trait itself. In a cultural setting, however, the survival of a patient rarely results directly in the dissemination of the medical procedure. While nutritional innovations, for instance, may directly benefit the innovator and her family, for most medical procedures the person who survives is rarely the person who invents or understands it. Medical evolution, therefore, depends upon the establishment and continuity, not of individuals but of social customs and institutions.

A second and equally important difference is that variation in Darwinian evolution is truly random, whereas cultural evolution has nonrandom elements. There is no intelligence, no mind at work to direct what variations arise in the evolution of biological species. The transmission of the adaptive trait is automatic, part of

189

a biologically programmed process of reproduction. Change is due to unpredictable mutations caused by uncontrollable environmental factors and the results are selected by natural processes. The fittest survive as a result of chance events, not intention.

Biorationalism makes medical evolution significantly different from Darwinian evolution. While medicine may have originated in random trial-and-error methods, it certainly could not have remained a random process for long because what was learned was remembered, taught, and analyzed. There are most definitely minds behind the selection process in medical evolution — inquisitive minds that pay attention to the hunter's chance of survival when white pus fills his wound; to the anomalous experience of the milkmaid who doesn't catch smallpox; to the surprising observation that the maggot-infested wounds of the soldier do not rot; to the reproductive histories of women who use cervical plugs of pomegranate or mud. Moreover, in cultural evolution, minds interact with other minds to transmit what is known and to *alter* behaviors. Men and women learn to vaccinate themselves against smallpox and do, they learn to prevent pregnancies and do. Thus people — and cultures — purposefully acquire characteristics that enhance their survival.

The selection process in medical evolution is therefore typical of Lamarckian rather than of Darwinian evolution. To cite Jean-Baptiste Lamarck in this day and age is sure to raise a furor, for his theory of evolution was discredited within the biological realm nearly a century ago, and with good reason. Lamarck essentially proposed that living things have a general tendency to improve and that the mechanism by which they do so is by striving to improve. The general theory is often called inheritance of acquired characteristics, for Lamarck assumed that any changes occurring in the physiognomy of an organism during its lifetime could be inherited. Thus he suggested that antelopes evolved into giraffes by constantly stretching their necks day after day in attempts to reach the leaves on ever-higher branches. We now know that, at least in higher animals, the germ-line cells that produce

190

egg and sperm are laid down prior to a person's birth and are not influenced by changes in physical makeup thereafter. No matter how many generations of Doberman pinschers have their tails cropped, they are still born with tails. No matter how many generations of Jews and Muslims are circumcised, their males are still born with a foreskin. Few people take Lamarck seriously anymore.

His ideas may still have their place, however, since cultural forms of evolution, such as that represented by the history of medicine, do involve the transmission of learned behavior. Whereas no multicellular organism that we know of can change its genetic structure during its lifetime in response to its natural environment or pass on environmentally induced alterations to its offspring, human behaviors and medical practices can and do change in response to their environment. The malleability of behavior and practice go hand in hand. There is no doubt that medicine improves because of the willful acquisition and retention of characteristics that confer improvement. There is no doubt that people change their medical behaviors and pass these changes on to others. This is, in fact, precisely the premise behind modern biomedical attempts to modify behaviors that affect health: don't eat high-cholesterol foods; eat more vegetables; don't smoke or drink when you are pregnant; do exercise. Not only does medical knowledge evolve in a Lamarckian manner, but the application of that knowledge unwittingly assumes the possibility of a Lamarckian evolution. What we do can affect our health and the health of our offspring as well. Culture does therefore influence biology as Lamarck suggested, even if it does not directly alter our genes.

Such insights into the evolutionary nature of medicine allow us to begin to say some things about the conditions under which medical progress is most likely to occur. For example, there is a geography to medical innovation, just as there is to biological evolution. In biological evolution, innovations tend to occur on the edges of large populations moving into new milieus or in small isolated populations that have adapted to unique environments. If

191

we look at where many of the medical innovations described in this book have occurred, they too have tended to be made in the geographical backwaters of medicine.

Withering and Jenner were private country doctors, not members of the medical faculty of some great university, nor were they even associated with any major hospital. The men who have reintroduced honey and sugar pastes into modern medicine, such as Martín in Ajoya, Mexico, Richard Knutson in a private clinic in Mississippi, and Leon Herszage in Buenos Aires, are obviously not major medical researchers at Harvard or Johns Hopkins or Stanford. Similarly, the many men who discovered and rediscovered cellophane bandages were all caught in unusual circumstances in isolated places where standard medical resources simply weren't available. Finally, it goes without saying that the folk medicines presently being investigated by pharmaceutical companies in New Guinea and other South Pacific islands, rural Africa and India, and the rain forests of South and Central America belong to medically isolated and conservative populations. That which is novel to the standards of Western medical culture must, by necessity, originate outside its purview.

An evolutionary perspective also allows us to understand the types of medicines that become integrated into standard medical practice from these geographically peripheral sources. Just as it is difficult for a new animal or plant species to arise in environments where well-adapted species already exist, so is it difficult for new medical treatments to arise where existing treatments are considered adequate or excellent. Medical evolution, like species evolution, only occurs when and where new niches open up. In biology, changes in climate or topography create new niches. In medicine, the recognition of unsolved problems, untreatable complications, and inadequate therapies creates new niches. So does the development of new resources, such as the chemistry to isolate novel compounds from plants, saliva, and urine, or the invention of new plastics and metal alloys. New medicines are likely to be found, not merely at the fringes of modern medicine, but at the juncture of persistent need and new or reappraised resources.

Innovation often requires not only a sense of frustration with standard medicines but a sense of urgency that liberates the physician from standard practice. Take, for example, the tendency of new medicine to rise from the ashes of catastrophe and war. The need to treat extraordinary cases in emergency rooms and trauma centers in times of war, or in areas where modern medical care is unavailable, gives healers tacit permission to experiment. During the Spanish Civil War severe shortages of standard medicaments, combined with overwhelming numbers of wounded men, forced surgeons like J. Trueta to extemporize with plaster casts and laudable pus. The technique worked so well it made inroads in peacetime medicine. The grim realities of civilian suffering and mortality can also fire medical creativity. Even with the best antibiotics available, chronic skin ulcers continue to bedevil thousands of patients, clearing the way for a resurgence of modernized treatments using maggots or sugar and honey. Because some forms of liver and kidney failure intractably resist pharmacological treatment, doctors are now giving the once reviled balneotherapy a second look. In each of these examples new advances have depended upon an inspirational return to the past.

Innovation does not always arise from planned revision, though. Sometimes it happens by chance, by serendipity. Just as nature sometimes creates unexpected and unusual hybrids among species, so it also throws together experiments that no scientist could imagine performing. The incidental folk observations that cowpox protects against smallpox were not planned. Nor was William Baer's first sight of a maggot-infested wound, but he marveled at what he saw with a thorough knowledge of the incurable nature of osteomyelitis and the dangers of gangrene. Covering burns with cellophane in an Italian POW camp began as an expedient to preclude worse forms of therapy, not to do any intrinsic good. These are examples of random associations, convergences of independent phenomena yielding results both unexpected and complementary. In each, nature did the work and spoke to someone who had the wisdom to listen. As Louis Pasteur said, "In the fields of observation chance favors only the prepared mind."

Medicine is also born of nonmedical needs and practices. It is often the case in biological evolution that so-called neutral mutations — those that confer neither an obvious advantage nor disadvantage — are the sources from which the most interesting novelties eventually arise. Honey, as we noted above, was probably first used simply because it felt good, not because it was believed to have healing properties. Similarly, taking the waters of Bath was pleasantly warm and soothing to the skin. And if an ill person said it made him feel better, well then, let him go on doing it. Therapies as innocuous as these could be used to treat almost any disease with some expectation that if they did not heal, at least they did not harm. This seems to be how yoga, meditation, massage, and other relaxation therapies are easing their way back into clinics today. And with time, patience, and many patients, perhaps a real effect, a real cure, may emerge.

What we have been describing is a process that evolutionary biologists call divergence: a variation that arises for one reason is modified to yield increasingly different innovations. The original primates evolved into monkeys, apes, and human beings, as an example. But just as there is divergence, there can also be convergence, the process by which different species in similar environments around the world evolve to look more and more similar. Anteaters, for example, are found in each of the major nonpolar continents. None of the different types is directly related, but all have evolved long, thin, sticky tongues, elongated noses, small eyes placed back on the head where ants will have difficulty finding and stinging them, and powerful front legs equipped with large claws for digging into ant nests.

Convergent evolution is also very apparent in medical evolution, although it is more likely to go under the name "simultaneous invention." Nearly every treatment described in this book developed independently in more than one culture, on more than one continent. Therapeutic practices involving honey, maggots, bathing, bloodletting, leeching, saliva, urine, clays, circumcision, contraception, and even cellophane exist all over the world. Some of these simultaneous medical inventions were similar or identical from culture to culture and remained so over extraordinarily long periods of time. Such persistence strongly suggests that given similar problems and similar materials, diverse peoples, just like adapting species, will converge on similar solutions by trial and error. When this happens, we can be reasonably certain that the result has some real survival value. Cross-cultural agreement on efficacy is therefore a useful standard of medical success.

In addition to divergence and convergence, there is another process at work in cultural evolution called dissociation. Sometimes nonmedical practices evolve from medical ones and become entirely independent. Circumcision is an example of a hygienic procedure that clearly has taken on mainly religious meanings for Jews and Muslims. Bathing, too, has diverse cultural meanings, as does bloodletting, variously used to dampen sexual urges, provide sacrifice for the gods, and affirm the lifelong friendship of blood brothers. Geophagy has also been subject to dissociation. The Tinggian of the Philippines, to cite one group with a history of eating earth in the distant past, today have a custom in which a newly married couple goes out into the fields. The husband places some earth on his axe, and he and his wife each eat some "so that," as the Tinggian say, "the ground will yield good harvests for them."

Condoms provide perhaps the most blatant example of dissociation between intended and actual use. Their original contraceptive use has, in many times and places, been superseded by their prophylactic use to inhibit the spread of venereal disease. In addition, they have been used as balloons, Christmas tree ornaments, covers for microphones for underwater use, and waterproof containers for innumerable small objects. During World War II, when all GIs were issued "rubbers," condoms were pulled over rifle barrels to keep them dry. In the recent Gulf War, American soldiers stretched condoms over the barrels of their firearms to keep out the sand. Drug smugglers fill condoms with cocaine and swallow them in order to pass through customs without getting caught. Dozens of other unintended uses undoubtedly exist. The point is, medical innovations such as the condom that depend on environmental resources for their invention and manufacture in turn add to those resources because of their invention. Medicine not only evolves within a general cultural milieu, it also changes that milieu by its very existence.

To summarize, medical traditions evolve just like species, adapting to local conditions such as plant life, mineral deposits, hot springs, and human technologies. People in every geographical locale try whatever is available to treat their indigenous diseases. Treatments that work survive and are modified by later generations. Cultures with access to similar resources and those that encounter similar medical problems rediscover similar efficacious treatments. Competition due to the gradual accumulation of medical knowledge tends to improve treatments over time, just as the accumulation of adaptive mutations tends to improve the adaptability of species over time.

The most important implication of this evolutionary view is that it focuses our attention on cross-cultural sources of new medical knowledge. Just as plant and animal hybrids are often strong and vigorous, due to the positive blending of characteristics selected from very different environments, so can the hybridization of medical traditions yield some of the most surprising and efficacious offspring. It is all a matter of creating enough variations within the context of stringent selection criteria. Under such conditions, something useful must result. Useful, therapeutic innovations, in turn, mean change. As medicine evolves within diverse cultures, it also alters them. It spins off unexpected nonmedical offspring. It becomes ritualized and stylized. The evolutionary dance is an intricate one, with all the complexities of a choreographed and orchestrated extravaganza. What makes it particularly exciting is that it is performed ad lib. We may be able to see the immediate step an innovation will take, but it is very rare that we foresee all the arabesques and pirouettes that may one day follow.

Our inability to foresee the future does not, however, prevent us from optimizing biorationalism in the present based on thousands of years of experience in the past. To do so, however, we must reexamine various aspects of the past, present, and future of medicine from an evolutionary perspective. First, how did medicine begin? Is mankind the first of living beings to practice medicine? Second, how can medicine best address the problems of a multicultural world in the future? If medicine evolves to fit specific niches, can any kind of medical therapy be appropriate and adequate to all cultures the world over? And third, how can we use evolutionary theory to help distinguish between the innovations of geniuses and the nonsense spread by crackpots and quacks? Indeed, why do patent nostrums and panaceas continue to plague the evolution of medicine? By looking both back and forward, as we shall do in the next three chapters, perhaps we can gain enough leverage on unnatural, cultural selection to guide the future course of medicine itself.

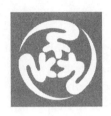

15.
APING THE APES

Man is a mammal and, like other animals, he is
equipped with instincts that drive him to commit
actions tending to preserve the individual. . . .
When illness has taken hold of the animal organism,
instincts manifest themselves in a special way. The
body craves what it needs to overcome the lesion and
restore health. The dog taken by a fever seeks rest
in a quiet corner, but is found eating herbs when his
stomach is upset. Nobody taught him what herbs to
eat, but he will instinctively seek those that make him
vomit or improve his condition in some other way.
. . . So man in illness craved and instinctively found
the other plants, animal parts, or minerals that his
body needed to overcome illness.

— Henry Sigerist, M.D., 1951

CHIMPS SHOW HUMANS NEW KIND OF
DRUG, read the 1991 newspaper head-
line. The story had actually begun in the mid-1980s while Harvard
University anthropologist Richard Wrangham, a protégé of Jane
Goodall, observed chimpanzees in Gombe National Park in Tanzania. For many years ethologists had heard tales from local peoples of monkeys and primates applying medicinal plants to
wounds or eating them when they were sick, but no scientist had
verified these legends. Wrangham, however, did. He observed that
chimps would often make special trips to find a type of sunflower

198

called *Aspilia,* characterized by tough, scratchy, and — as Wrangham found out for himself — virtually inedible leaves. The chimps sometimes chewed these leaves and on certain occasions swallowed several of them whole.

Subsequent studies revealed two very interesting things about these leaves. First, they contain an oil called thiarubrine-A that kills many types of bacteria, fungi, and parasitic worms. By swallowing the leaves whole, the chimps probably deliver a therapeutic amount of the oil to the gut, where it can combat intestinal ailments. Second, *Aspilia* has long been used by people in Tanzania for similar ailments. The combination of animal and human use led scientists to explore the nature of thiarubrine-A further and they found that it has significant anticancer activity as well.

It should not astonish us that apes or even other mammals seem to dose themselves with the same medicinal plants used in human folk medicines. Physiologically we are almost identical to our primate cousins. And psychologically and socially there are many similarities, too. Ethologist Desmond Morris considers human beings nothing more than "naked apes." His not-too-subtle point is that, much as we would like to consider ourselves substantially superior to the rest of creation, we are still animals. We are linked to other mammals not only in our physical evolution but in our behavioral evolution as well. We have the same sexual urges, the same desires for food, comfort, cleanliness, and companionship. We also have the same urge to relieve discomfort, pain, and suffering. Indeed, human health rituals differ only in scale, not in kind, from those of our mammalian cousins.

For example, like all animals we groom ourselves and each other to remove ticks, fleas, and other pests. Soldiers serving in tropical areas will cover their faces and hands with mud to protect themselves against mosquitoes and gnats, just as other animals will roll in mud holes or bogs or cover themselves in dust to discourage the pests. Where that is not appropriate, we have invented artificial tails (which we call fans and fly swatters) to keep flying and biting insects away. Henry Sigerist, medical historian and doctor, has even gone so far as to suggest that the scratching of animals has been altered by human beings into scarification, the sucking and licking of wounds has developed into cupping, and the instinctive rubbing of an injured limb has become our massage.

Credibility may be stretched rather far by the ancient Greek claim that human bloodletting began when a man observed a sick hippopotamus purposefully cut itself on some sharp stakes; nevertheless, the possibility of animal phlebotomy is intriguing. There are eighteenth-century reports of deer and goats relieving their pain by inducing bleeding near infected sites. Sigerist argues that among humans "bleeding as a method of treatment was so universal that it also must be derived from instinctive actions. . . . Individuals suffering from fever diseases suddenly felt relieved when they had a spontaneous hemorrhage, bleeding from the nose or when menstruation set in." Animals, too, can feel the spontaneous relief of hemorrhage, independent of the ability to act purposefully upon their experience and let blood. Some forms of experience, however, they can manipulate. Many of the treatments discussed in this book were, in fact, pioneered for humanity by other animals and are still used by them today. Aping the apes can have its benefits, and therein lies an important clue to the origins of human medicine and to its future.

To understand the behavioral roots from which medicine evolved, there is no better way to start than by watching our fellow animals. This is not to say that apes or other animals "know" that what they do is medically useful, but the physiological and psychological drives that we associate with therapeutic intent in humans may very well have infrahuman origins. Modern Nigerians still frequent a salt lick near Lake Chad to procure *kanwa,* an earth used as a nutritional supplement — and so do the local animals. In neither case is therapeutic intention necessary for physiological benefit. Indeed, primitive peoples who added clay to their wild potatoes or acorn mash could not have known why it worked. What they did know is that the mixture tasted better because it was not so bitter. Similarly, no one before this century could possibly have understood why licking wounds helped them to heal, how

honey fought infection, or why head-out immersion actually relieved dropsy or lead palsy. The science simply did not exist. But
people partaking of these therapies felt better, and so could animals who did similar things. When feeling better correlated with
increased probability of survival, then the behavior was adaptive
and evolution selected for it. "Try it and see" sometimes became
"do it and live" among animals as well as people. Survival became
tied not just to genes but to culture.

One thing is certain: some human medicines have evolved
from the imitation of animals. As recently as forty years ago the
native healers of Ponape, one of the eastern Caroline Islands in
the South Pacific, were still paying serious attention to the symptoms and behavior of sick animals. If an animal ate a particular
plant and recovered, then people with apparently similar symptoms tried it, too. Investigators at Shaman Pharmaceuticals have
observed a similar attentiveness to animal physic among native
healers in other parts of the world. By the same token, native
healers in Samoa test new treatments by feeding them to dogs or
pigs before they try them on people.

The rise of animal husbandry may have promoted further
medical learning useful to human beings. For many generations,
for example, American Indian women in what is now the United
States drank an infusion of the roots of stoneweed, *Lithospermum
ruderale,* as a contraceptive. Most chroniclers of this practice wrote
it off as superstition. But when a "plague of sterility," as local
ranchers called it, struck cattle in the midwestern states during the
1950s, it was eventually traced to the animals' ingestion of an herb
known to Indians as desert tea — another name for *Lithospermum.*
Subsequent laboratory research on mice, rats, and rabbits confirmed that the root and alcoholic extracts of the plant did indeed
abolish normal estrus by interfering with the hormones that control reproduction. Whether the Indians discovered the contraceptive effects of *Lithospermum* by trial and error or, as modern investigators did, by observing its effects on domestic or wild animals
must, of course, remain conjectural.

Though causality cannot be proved in every case, Calvin

Schwabe, an expert on the history of medicine, has argued that much of formalized ancient medicine did depend upon the domestication of animals. In learning to raise healthy animals, people also learned what was necessary to maintain their own health. He finds, for example, many notable similarities between the treatments used by ancient Egyptians for their cattle and those they used on themselves. Animals became the model for humans long before modern science had ever conceived of the discipline of pharmacology or of animal testing protocols and FDA regulations. What is healthful for animals is often (though not always) healthful for us.

Certainly, anyone who watches animals closely must be struck by the similarities between some of their therapeutic behaviors and human medicine. Consider the habit of licking wounds: dogs, cats, rats, mice, rabbits, guinea pigs, and many other mammals frequently lick their own wounds and sometimes those of others. We vividly remember observing a college friend's dog develop an eye infection that continuously oozed pus. Another dog would come by several times a day to lick its friend's eye, and sure enough, in a matter of days the eye infection was gone.

The urge to lick is so strong in some animals that the care can even be carried across species. James Herriot observed a farm dog named Judy, who carried the caring habit to such extremes that she seems to have had what one might call a nursing complex. On one occasion, when Herriot had given a bull an injection, Judy watched carefully and then licked the bull's neck methodically at the injection site. She stayed with the bull all night, licking him occasionally, until it was clear he would recover. She would also lick each newborn calf, helping the mother do her maternal duty. And one time she even tried to adopt — and lick — a brood of newborn chicks!

The habit of licking wounds exists in our closest evolutionary cousins as well. Dian Fossey recorded that injured gorillas will clean any wounds they can reach with hands or tongue. Whether intentionally or not, such grooming keeps the wound clean, irrigated, constantly supplied with salivary antibiotics, and open for drainage of pus. Sometimes gorillas will even treat each other. Fossey watched a young female caring for her mother, Effie, who had been severely injured during an encounter with a neighboring gorilla group.

> Within a week her bite wounds were draining badly and, had it not been for Effie's five-year-old daughter Tuck, the injuries would have taken far longer to heal than they did. Tuck appointed herself Effie's attentive and almost overzealous groomer, pushing away other animals who interfered with her ministrations. Tuck even pushed away the hands of Effie, who, possibly because of discomfort, wanted only to be left alone. Tuck licked and probed stubbornly at the bite injuries until all had healed six weeks after their infliction.

In a less successful case, a gorilla that had broken free of a trap had wire embedded in her leg. Although Lee, the injured gorilla, and her mother, Petula, groomed the wound regularly for three months, Lee eventually died of gangrene and pneumonia. Nevertheless, to have survived such a wound for three months in the jungle without any "modern" medicines is hardly a failure; rather it testifies to the relative efficacy of such simple therapies.

Chimpanzees also lick themselves and each other for a variety of health-related purposes. Jane Goodall has noted that chimps, like almost all land-living mammals, immediately lick and groom their newborns. Chimps also tend to "lick their wounds if these are on hands or feet or other easily accessible parts. Or they may repeatedly touch the lesion with their fingers, which they then lick. Often they dab the wound with a handful of leaves, which are then usually sniffed and dropped, but may be licked and reused. Infants and juveniles have been seen to lick their mother's wounds, but an adult usually grooms carefully around the wound of a companion — though he may stare at it intently."

Urine, too, seems to be part of the health-care regimens of various animals. Capuchin and squirrel monkeys as well as lorises

in South America habitually urinate into their hands and then rub
the urine over their feet and fur. The function of this habit is still
the subject of great controversy, since it is not clear whether the
urine cools the animals when they become too hot, acts as a sexual
attractant, marks territory as they move about, or plays some other
role. One suggestion that has not, apparently, been investigated is
that urine washing in monkeys, as in man, keeps the fur and skin
soft and healthy. Given the antiseptic actions of urea, urine washing might also help prevent fungal and other infections and remove insects and pests — no small problem in the jungle.

Animals also drink urine. Pigs, for example, will ingest each
other's urine if they are malnourished or ill. So will chimpanzees,
who even drink human urine when they find it. Many domesti-
cated animals have been observed doing the same — perhaps ex-
plaining the "taste" dogs and some cats seem to have for toilet
bowls! As far as we can determine, however, no one documenting
urine drinking among animals has considered the possibility that
it might be therapeutic, probably because the medicinal benefits
for humans have been so little appreciated.

Many animals also practice geophagy, which seems to play as
many diverse roles for them as it does for humans. Eating soil,
mud, clay, and even rocks is not only a common, but sometimes an
essential, component of animal nutrition. Animals, too, require
minerals such as calcium, iron, potassium, magnesium, phosphorus, selenium, and zinc. They also require salt. Despite the bad
press today for sodium chloride, too little can be as debilitating as
too much. When animals are deficient in salts or minerals, they
find ways to supplement their diets. In fact, the drive to do so is so
intense among some species that the locations of nutritive earths
became plentiful hunting grounds for early man. The bones of
extinct mammoths are often found beside prehistoric salt licks.

When wild animals are kept in captivity, it is often necessary
to cater to their natural geophagy. Animal keepers at the Baltimore Zoo in the 1950s provided their kangaroos with three or
four pounds of red clay each week as a dietary supplement to

keep them healthy. In fact, the keepers regularly offered many mammals clumps of grass with earth clinging to the roots and observed that the animals ate the clumps whole, dirt and all. Animals provided with such dietary supplements had healthier coats than those who were not.

Animals in the wild may also use clays medicinally. Experiments on laboratory rats have shown that they will ingest clay if they develop gastrointestinal distress. And primatologist William Mahaney of York University, Ontario, thinks that gorillas in the Virunga Mountains of Rwanda may eat some types of clay for their antidiarrheal activity, rather than for their mineral content, which is low. These clays contain a great deal of halloysite, a highly binding clay related to kaolin. Mahaney suggests that the gorillas "may use halloysite as the equivalent of a pharmaceutical drug to offset or cure diarrhea which is often epidemic among different gorilla groups." If this is true, then gorillas, and possibly other mammals as well, had probably found a natural Kaopectate long before the modern drug industry even existed!

Some investigators have conjectured that geophagy in animals such as the monkeys and great apes has less to do with mineral deficiencies or disease than it does with detoxifying alkaloids and tannins in the fruits, nuts, and leaves that make up much of their diet. As Timothy Johns points out, "Clay eating provides the consumer with a certain degree of protection, allowing greater flexibility of choice in the diet — an especially important adaptation in times of famine. That many animals, including chimpanzees and gorillas, regularly eat clay supports the idea that the detoxifying effects of clay eating confer an evolutionary advantage."

Whatever the reasons, the great apes certainly do make soil part of their regular diet. Although gorillas get most of their nutrition from plants, about 10 percent of their diet consists, according to Dian Fossey, of "dung, dirt, bark, roots, grubs and snails." Soil-eating binges occur periodically, especially during the dry season when other food often grows scarce. Each gorilla group has its favorite "dig." One group likes sandy slides; another, rich forest soil abundant in calcium and potassium. Fossey found that a location favored by one of the groups she studied

> had been so dug out by the gorillas that the tree roots formed exposed gnarled supports for the vast caves created by the animals' repeated soil digging. . . . It was eerie to watch the huge silverback magically disappear beneath the web of tree roots into total blackness. When he emerged, covered with the sandy crumbs of his feast, he moved off, leaving the cave to the other group members. In order of rank, they disappeared into its depths. Their subsequent screams and pig-grunts reflected the overcrowded conditions.

Most other primates include earths in their cuisines as well. Japanese macaques regularly eat soil, but whether for nutrition or the antidiarrheal effects remains unclear. Some chimps and many baboons have been observed to lick rocks lying in streambeds or beside lakes. Goodall has reported seeing chimpanzees repeatedly eat soil from a cliff face at Gombe that baboons, bushbucks, and various birds also frequent. Just as some gorillas have burrowed caves as a result of their mineral mining, the chimps and other animals have gouged hollows in the cliff faces. Goodall also reports that "about once a day [the chimps at Gombe] pause to pick off and eat small amounts [of termite clay] — not more than would fill a walnut . . . as they pass termite mounds." As noted previously with regard to human consumption of ant and termite clays — a habit that may have originated either by imitation of apes or in our hominid prehistory — chimps may benefit from "potassium, magnesium, and calcium and traces of copper, manganese, zinc, and sodium" in the termite earth — a veritable mineral supplement pill!

Our nearest cousins have found evolutionary advantages in bathing, too. Although most adult apes and monkeys avoid water and cannot swim, young rhesus and macaque monkeys often play in it. Such play is in evidence among groups of Japanese macaques that patronize hot springs on cold mornings or snowy winter days,

206

where they sit or swim for thirty minutes or so. The behavior clearly conserves their energy by keeping them warm. Conversely, macaques in tropical regions seem to use bathing to avoid the heat or simply to play. Whatever the reasons, the amount of time spent by these monkeys in head-out immersion is, in fact, sufficient to produce the same renal and vascular changes that are experienced by human beings (and monkeys) under clinical conditions.

Actually, primate bathing sheds some intriguing light on the animal behaviors that we have found to be medically beneficial. Their origins may be rooted both in play and in survival. In either case, primate bathing also makes clear that such therapeutic behaviors are not necessarily "natural." Monkeys learn bathing and swimming habits from each other. Only certain groups partake in these activities or invent them for themselves. Bathing among primates has the definite characteristics of culture rather than instinct.

Other primate behaviors with medical benefits may be cultural as well. Amazingly enough, monkeys have been known to use honeylike substances for treating their wounds. In 1987 G. Westergaard of the University of Washington and Dorothy Fragaszy of Washington State University reported that a captive capuchin monkey named Alice learned to modify a stick in order to obtain maple-flavored corn syrup from a closed container with only a small hole for access. Fifty-six days later Alice acquired a cut on her finger. Over the next few days she was observed repeatedly preparing a stick by biting and feathering its end, dipping it into the syrup and applying it to her wound. We may assume that the syrup made the wound feel better, as has been reported by human beings using honey and sugar salves. Alice used the syrup on three subsequent lesions over the next few months. One of these was large enough to require five stitches. Alice carefully removed them with a stick and self-treated with her syrup several times a day. Like all of her wounds, this one healed completely, without infection or complication.

So far, the use of honey to treat wounds has not been observed in the wild. However, wild chimpanzees regularly "fish" for honey from nests built by both stinging and stingless species of bees. Special sticks similar to those made by Alice are often prepared for these honey hunting forays and used both to swat at the bees and to probe the nests. In one case a young female chimpanzee was observed making a tool set of sticks of varying sizes and thicknesses in order to complete a successful honey-fishing expedition. It would take only a bit of honey on an open cut on this chimp's hand for a wild connection between injury and remedy to emerge.

This is not as conjectural as it may seem. We now know, without any doubt, that it does not take a human mind to make such discoveries or to apply them. There have been other "Alices" among the wild primates, just as there have been many human "Alices." The origins of human medicine are deeply embedded in habits such as honey hunting that were acquired long ago in our evolutionary past.

Alice the capuchin monkey also provides us with possible insights into the origins of surgery. A year after she experimented with syrup for wound treatment, her infant sustained major head injuries following an apparent attempt at infanticide by one or more members of Alice's group. The infant's skull was fractured, and broken fragments of bone were embedded in the brain. Alice attempted to clean the wound using both fingers and her mouth (thus applying saliva). When these methods proved ineffectual, she prepared a stick by chewing one end to form a soft, brush-like edge. She then attempted to "sweep" the debris from the wound. The infant was subsequently taken from its mother and given veterinary treatment, but it died of infection. One interpretation of Alice's behavior is that having learned to make tools, she quickly applied them to new situations, such as the treatment of injuries. Chimpanzees have made the same leap, occasionally probing open wounds with small sticks. Again, it is reasonable to assume that primitive human beings would have behaved in similar ways and that surgery — which has often been called the oldest form of medicine — may have originated along with tool use.

Apes and monkeys have, in fact, been observed carrying out

a wide range of what we would characterize in human settings as simple medical, surgical, and even dental practices. At one zoo a female chimpanzee was observed approaching a male and whimpering. The male, Desmond Morris tells us, "took her head gently but firmly in his left hand and started to pull down her left lower eyelid with his right forefinger. Peering intently at her left eye, he searched her eyelid and eventually located a small cinder that had lodged there. With extreme delicacy he removed it." As Morris notes, these actions hardly differ from what might be expected of a pair of human beings.

Suffering from severe nasal congestion, another chimp named Kalunde learned that he could make himself sneeze and thereby clear his nasal passages by putting a small stick up his nose. If this activity sounds bizarre, consider that human beings have, at various times and places, used pepper, snuff, and other irritants for similar purposes. While the origin of the chimpanzee behavior was not observed, it is suspected that Kalunde may have accidentally discovered the "treatment" while fishing for ants with a long, thin stick he had recently made for that purpose. Kalunde used his stick to induce sneezing only while his congestion was especially severe.

Chimpanzees have also been seen using plant fibers and small sticks to extract material stuck between their teeth, just as we use dental floss and toothpicks. While most chimps use these tools on themselves, Goodall repeatedly observed a female chimpanzee named Belle using twigs to clean the teeth of other troop members. Belle even tried to help a number of her peers extract their loose "baby" teeth and on one occasion succeeded. Anthropological studies suggest that such dental grooming may have been one of the oldest and most widespread practices of early humans. Grooves in teeth consistent with regular use of toothpicks have been found in skulls of *Homo habilis* dating to 1.84 million years ago, and many examples exist of *Homo erectus* and *Homo sapiens* skulls with similar grooves from the period 130,000 to 70,000 years ago. Evidence for this kind of dental care is continuous up until the present and across cultures as diverse as paleolithic cave dwellers, Australian aborigines, Canary Islanders, ancient Egyptians, and American Indians.

Perhaps the most stunning observation of all is that some monkeys may have found natural ways to control when they enter estrus. Primatologist Karen Strier of the University of Wisconsin at Madison has found that during nonreproductive periods muriqui monkeys in Brazil tend to eat large amounts of plants that contain fertility-reducing estrogen mimics called isoflavonoids. They switch to a diet high in plants having steroid compounds that promote fertility when they are ready to mate. Again, the issue is not whether the monkeys "understand" what they are doing but rather whether our prehuman and prehistoric ancestors may have, knowingly or not, begun to regulate their own reproductive capacities in similar ways. Notably, the area of South America in which these monkeys live is the same in which some primitive tribes still use plant compounds for birth control. Again it appears that it may not take a human mind to take medicinal advantage of the chance effects of environmental agents. If the behavior is beneficial and becomes habitual, if it can be learned or imitated, then it can affect evolution.

Now for the punchline. If we are but naked apes, and if we share so much of both our physiology and our medical heritage with our mammalian cousins, then it is only logical to presume that we can look not only to our own folklore and customs for medical enlightenment, but to the therapeutic practices of other animals as well. This, in fact, is the premise behind zoopharmocognosy, coined from the Greek root words *zōo, pharmakon,* and *gnōsis* and meaning "animal pharmaceutical knowledge." Indeed, ethological medicine has as many hidden surprises for modern medical practice as has ethnomedicine.

The notion that humans can learn important things about medicine from watching animals is no longer the mere speculation it was when Wrangham first observed chimps eating *Aspilia* leaves at Gombe. It has now entered the realm of practice. At least two other, well-documented instances demonstrate that apes use plants known by humans to have medicinal properties. Toshisada

Nishida and Paul Newton have observed sick chimpanzees chewing a variety of leaves used in human herbal remedies. Similarly, J. Phillips-Conroy has noted that when baboons develop schistosomiasis, caused by a parasitic worm, they alter their diet to ingest plants with deworming chemical components. These and other cases have led Eloy Rodriguez, a professor of environmental sciences at Cornell University, to suggest that pharmaceutical companies would benefit by observing how apes and monkeys in the wild use medicinal plants. In other words, we should imitate those primitive healers on Ponape who watch the animals for clues to new treatments. If his approach catches on, the old saying "Monkey see, monkey do" may become the basis of a new, and quite serious, monkey business.

This business will be quite a change from the laboratory use of animals that has become a hallmark of human medical experimentation. For people who have qualms about the testing of human medical therapies on captive animals, the idea that free, wild animals may teach us useful medical practices of their own volition should be welcome. By drawing upon ethological sources for new medicines, human beings learn from animals who have willingly experimented upon themselves.

For evolutionists as well there must be a certain satisfaction in being able to say that we are not beyond learning from the apes. If anyone needs a purely pragmatic reason for conserving both the indigenous lands and the indigenous populations of wild animals that are threatened by extinction around the globe, zoopharmacognosy and ethological medicine provide it. Every group of gorillas, chimpanzees, monkeys, elephants, or other social mammals that is destroyed carries with it another ten or hundred million years of experimental knowledge. This is knowledge that could benefit not only human beings but other animals as well through ethology-based veterinary care — a field that we have not even begun to explore.

It may do our pride some harm to sit before the apes like children and ask to be taught, but it will do our intellect much good.

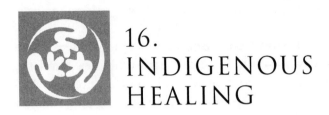

16.
INDIGENOUS
HEALING

*Just as America was considered to be undiscovered
before the white men found it, so the Indian drugs
were unreal or of no account until white men
discovered them. This is one example among many
of the ethnocentric attitude which has hurt the white
men more than the Indian by delaying scientific
inquiry into aboriginal herbal knowledge.*

— Virgil Vogel, Ph.D., 1970

W HEN ANTHROPOLOGIST Laura Bohannan left Oxford to live with the Tiv
tribe in Africa, she took along a copy of Shakespeare's *Hamlet,* a
gift from a friend. During the long, wet season in which her Tiv
acquaintances were almost completely indolent, she spent many
long hours alone pondering the meaning of the play. After nearly
two months of study, she was certain not only that she understood
Shakespeare's meaning but that there was only one universal interpretation of it.

A few weeks later Bohannan got a chance to find out if she
was right. All of the male elders of the tribe had gathered in a hut
to drink their homemade beer, chew cola nuts, and tell stories.
Disturbed that they had seen so little of her, they asked why she
spent so much time with her "paper" — their word for all things
written. Bohannan replied that it was a famous story of her ancestors. The Tiv demanded that she tell it.

It is impossible to do justice in a few sentences to Bohannan's classic article "Shakespeare in the Bush," in which she describes her subsequent trials and tribulations, but a few illustrations will provide the flavor of her narrative. Her problems began as soon as she mentioned the appearance of the ghost of Hamlet's father. The Tiv do not believe in an afterlife and therefore have no concept of ghosts. Their closest equivalent is an omen sent by a witch, so of course they wanted to know which witch was involved. Her explanation that the ghost came of its own accord simply demonstrated to the Tiv elders that Bohannan did not understand the story. When she added that the ghost actually spoke to Hamlet and walked with him, they were simply incredulous: omens can't speak and dead men can't walk.

The Tiv were confirmed in their impression that Bohannan was terribly confused when she tried to explain that Hamlet was upset by the fact that his mother had married his father's brother less than a month after the funeral. The European outrage that one brother would kill another to take power and consolidate it by marriage with his sister-in-law was incomprehensible to them. If a husband dies in their culture, it is the obligation of the younger brother to marry the widow and become father to his brother's children, and the sooner the better. In their view the villain of Shakespeare's play had acted quite properly.

It was all downhill from there. The Tiv had no concept of mental illness, so Hamlet's breakdown was inexplicable. Moreover, his attempt to revenge his father, which Europeans accept as understandable behavior, the Tiv considered aberrant because it was not their way for sons to avenge fathers, but for the father's peers to do so. Hamlet, they felt, was stepping out of line. Suffice it to say, Bohannan left the elders' hut that morning quite convinced that Shakespeare — and human behavior — was not as universally comprehensible as she had believed. Indeed, the most senior of the Tiv elders asked Bohannan to tell them more Western stories in the future so that they could instruct her in their true meanings.

It is worth thinking about Bohannan's story in the context of medicine. Each culture, including our own, naturally assumes that its ways are the best and most appropriate model for the rest of the world. Sophisticated modern medicines work best for us, so there is no reason, we believe, they should not work best for everyone else. We must recognize, however, that because medicine is a form of culture, it is as open to alternative interpretations and uses as is *Hamlet* in the hands of the Tiv. The history of medicine is full of examples of non-Europeans resisting European medicine, sometimes with very good reason.

For example, numerous attempts by authorities in North America to variolize and later vaccinate Indians against smallpox met with considerable resistance in the eighteenth and nineteenth centuries. Not surprisingly, many tribes suspected the Europeans' intentions — in some cases properly so, since there is clear-cut evidence that some Europeans deliberately did spread smallpox to kill Indians. Even when the white men meant well, however, their efforts were often misunderstood. The refusal of many Indians to submit to vaccination hinged on their perceptions of what medicine should and should not be. In the early nineteenth century George Catlin, renowned for his portraits of North American Indians, remarked that they found it hard to accept that a small puncture in the arm could protect them from a fatal disease. In fact, as a trader's clerk in the Upper Missouri observed, they often believed that inoculation was far more likely to produce harm than good: "Should any accident happen or should the Indian miss his hunt, or any casualty befall him or his family, the vaccination would be blamed for it." True medicine, for most tribes, involved the spiritual readjustment of the individual to his clan, his environment, and his gods, not just a mechanical manipulation of the body or its symptoms. Thus few Indians submitted to the suspicious procedure of vaccination except when actual smallpox outbreaks occurred. White men had not learned that medicines need to be more than just efficacious, they must also be delivered in forms that are consonant with cultural belief.

Cultural refusals of Western medicine continue to this day in other areas of the world. In Ethiopia, for example, porphyria cutanea tarda related to alcohol abuse occurs in 2 percent or more of the population. Porphyria cutanea tarda, recall, is one of the few diseases for which Western medicine prescribes phlebotomy as the preferred and optimal treatment. Regular, copious bloodletting reduces the accumulation of porphyrins and the iron overload that often accompanies the disease. The Ethiopians, nonetheless, categorically refuse to be phlebotomized. Blood is not let for anything but the most sacrosanct ceremonial reasons. In any case, because the bleedings must be done repeatedly over a long period of time this treatment is inappropriate for a population that visits health-care facilities only transiently and from long distances. Physicians have learned that a single ten-day treatment with the antimalarial drug chloroquine is both efficacious and acceptable for this population. Unfortunately, chloroquine carries a risk of long-term damage to the liver, a trade-off that must be made to prevent death from porphyria.

The Ethiopian abhorrence of bloodletting is really not that hard for us to understand. It is equally apparent, though of different origins, in the refusal of Christian Scientists and Seventh-day Adventists in the United States to accept medical treatments involving blood or materials derived from blood. In fact, most of us would probably rather take a pill than open a vein, but chloroquine is not optimal medicine, and we find the better treatment acceptable. The drawing of blood is so much a part of our regular medical check-ups that we recognize phlebotomy as an appropriate therapeutic tool. Thus our own medical and cultural beliefs dictate how we wish to be treated just as they dictate acceptable treatments in other parts of the world.

Medicine's "fit" or lack of fit with diverse cultural niches is perhaps best-documented by the fortunes of birth control. In medieval Islam, for example, withdrawal did not violate religious principles because man's acts of contraception, which failed an appreciable amount of the time, were never more powerful than divine purpose. Coitus interruptus was a primary form of birth control in that culture. Within the Jewish tradition, however, any form of contraception that interfered with or harmed the male sperm could not be condoned and coitus interruptus was forbidden.

Coitus interruptus was also forbidden for European Christians, but for very different reasons. Christian notions of the divine purpose of intercourse made that religion highly critical of nonreproductive sex or of any interference with the natural course of conception. Sex purely for pleasure was especially sinful, so coitus interruptus was unacceptable on several grounds. The Christian and Judaic hostility to this and other forms of contraception has lasted for many centuries. Yet when appropriate contraception was discovered or developed — that is, contraception that did not violate particular religious beliefs — these techniques were readily adopted by both religious cultures. In 1951 the Catholic Church approved the rhythm method, a contraceptive technique that does not interfere with natural reproductive processes. With the development of the pill, orthodox Judaism also found an appropriate contraceptive, one that did not harm the male sperm.

The same social and economic forces that created an environment for widespread contraceptive use in Western culture over the past two hundred years are at work today throughout the Third World. Emerging nations in the early stages of economic industrialization commonly gain mastery over the major causes of death — death control — well before mastery over rates of birth. Declining mortality, coupled with unregulated high fertility, spur tremendous population growth that stalls further economic development. Yet even when the need or desire for birth control is recognized, Western contraceptive technologies have not always been accepted because of religious beliefs, issues of body image, sexual taboos, and perceived risks.

In Bangladesh, for example, the predominantly Islamic population has resisted modern birth control methods because of the traditional importance of purdah, the pious seclusion of women that enhances social respectability. In countries where many women still engage in public laundering of menstrual rags, any change in the menstrual cycle is a pronouncement about one's sexual life. Intercourse is often forbidden during menstruation, so a long period keeps a woman from her conjugal duties. A short period or its absence provokes speculation that she is pregnant. For many Bangladeshis the body is the physical representation of one's moral and social life. Unfortunately, the pill and injectable contraceptives such as Depo-Provera can cause irregular menstruation, particularly during the initial months of use, which the women of Bangladesh consider a sign of bad health — precisely because it disrupts their traditional pious behavior. We in the West take our sexual privacy so much for granted that it is difficult for us to appreciate the extent to which the acceptability of birth control is affected by public constraints upon behavior.

Body image and sexual taboos also act to promote or demote the use of particular contraceptive techniques. Vasectomy, or male sterilization, is the method of choice in Korea, and condoms the method of choice in Singapore and Japan. Indeed, the Japanese account for one quarter of condom users worldwide. A strong sexual inhibition among traditional Asian women that includes a dislike of handling their genitals has led these cultures to rely almost exclusively on male contraception. The situation is dramatically different in Jamaica where some women fear that condoms will fall off and rot in the womb and for this reason have resisted their use. Women in Peru object to condoms because they are thought to cause pimples on the face. They also avoid the pill for fear that they will give birth to monsters. Rhythm is the Peruvian method of choice, in keeping with the country's Catholic roots. In contrast, in African countries where scarification is practiced, contraceptive implants are well received, presumably because the surgical procedure is consistent with existing ritual. Injectables are popular where vaccination has already gained ground.

All in all, efficacy has almost nothing to do with the types of birth control any particular culture finds acceptable. In order to be practiced, birth control must comply with certain social standards in general, such as ease of use and lack of medical or nuisance side effects, but also with local customs, religious beliefs, and sexual taboos. A people cannot be treated without reference to their culture.

From an evolutionary perspective, this coadaptation between general culture and medical treatment is not only understandable but necessary. Medical species, just like biological species, must adapt to their environment. The best treatment is not simply the most efficacious one, but the one that is actually put to use. Use, in turn, may depend on cultural beliefs and taboos, the availability of medical resources, or pure economics. !Kung bushmen in the Kalahari Desert or starving peasants in rural Bangladesh might benefit from having an intensive-care unit, but the fact is that they must make do with other medical measures. That which is considered best or most adaptive or most efficacious can be determined only in relation to a complex environment comprising economic, social, technological, intellectual, and cultural factors.

If we look back at the various treatments discussed in this book, the manner in which these factors affect medicine becomes eminently clear. Consider, for example, how the reemergence of honey and sugar treatments at Project Projimo in Ajoya, Mexico, illustrates the importance of the economic niche. The healer Martín was constrained in his choice of treatments by four major issues: lack of medical facilities, relative availability of drugs and other therapeutic agents, their cost, and their relative effectiveness. The local economic environment would not support the expensive, high-tech antibiotic and surgical treatments that are preferred in well-to-do, industrialized areas. Wound care had to be locally accessible and economically feasible, whether provided by healer, clinic, or hospital. And, of course, it had to be medically effective. Honey fit all these requirements, even more than sugar, because it alone was universally available.

Economic viability has also been an issue for physicians treating burns in underdeveloped areas of the world. And again honey has been widely adopted in parts of India and Africa where, as in Ajoya, cost prohibits the use of high-tech medicines. An even more striking example of economic influence on treatment choice can

218

be found in the medical use of cellophane. As we have learned, cellophane bandages were invented almost as soon as the technology for producing the plastic was made generally available. Expense and the lack of an obvious need for new bandages initially stymied their development, but eventually their reinvention during World War II led to a whole new breed of high-tech wound coverings. At the time, only highly industrialized countries (or their colonies) directly benefited from these developments. High-tech plastics were and still are too expensive for the majority of the world's people.

Ironically, the need for an inexpensive, effective *alternative* to plastic bandages such as Opsite and its cousins recently led to a third round of cellophane rediscovery. In 1991, nearly fifty years after the heyday of cellophane bandaging, a group of five physicians in the Burn Research Unit of the Bai Jerbai Wadia Hospital for Children in Bombay, India, reported the "novel" observation that cellophane was a good substitute material for treating wounds associated with burn treatment. Like most physicians treating burns in this modern age, Dr. Vartak and his colleagues transplanted skin from unaffected parts of the body to help cover the burned area, a procedure that necessarily creates a second wound in healthy tissue. Like so many of his predecessors, Vartak found that the daily changing of standard paraffin-impregnated gauze bandages at these donor sites caused such extreme pain that anesthesia was often required. While appreciative of the more sophisticated synthetic and biological membranes such as Opsite, Vartak noted that even these caused some pain, and "their prohibitive cost prevents their routine use in our country."

Apparently unaware of the medical uses of cellophane in the 1930s and '40s, Vartak and his colleagues rode the wheel of invention around in a circle. "Cellophane paper was thought of because of its similarity in appearance with Opsite and other similar dressings. It is very cheap and easily available in stationery shops all over this country. . . . A dressing of the donor area involving one adult thigh (skin graft obtained from about 4 per cent of body surface area) costs about one rupee (30 rupees = 1 £ sterling =

US $2). It can be sterilized by conventional autoclaving and does not need any special equipment." In addition to these economic and technical advantages, Vartak's group found (again like their unsuspected predecessors) that cellophane was easy to work with. Once it was in place, it rarely needed to be replaced, and it sloughed off easily as new skin grew beneath it. No patient in the study complained of pain when his or her wound was covered with cellophane, nor did any of the wounds become infected. All in all, this reemergence of cellophane bandaging can be considered a species of treatment that nearly went extinct, then reevolved in a new place where "more advanced" species could not survive the local economic conditions due to availability and cost.

Treatments can also come into being or die out for reasons that have to do with their social niche. Such is the case with the British history of smallpox variolization and vaccination. In the early 1700s Lady Mary Wortley Montagu had convinced the royal family to be inoculated with weakened smallpox material, and average citizens had followed suit. In turn, the acceptance of this procedure presented a severe obstacle to Jenner's safer, more efficacious cowpox vaccine later in the century. By that time British society was tied by habit and vested interest to variolization; medical practitioners had founded not only individual careers but whole institutions based upon the procedure. Fortunately, Jenner had made the acquaintance of many lords and ladies taking the waters at Cheltenham, including, too, members of the royal family. He used these fashionable connections to spread his own innovation. Once Jenner convinced key members of the aristocracy that vaccination was better than variolization, he found, as Lady Wortley Montagu had, that other people began to listen as well. Fashion dictated not only clothing and manners but medical treatments.

Fashions in medicine, which represent nothing more than the persuasive spread of a social niche, can also die out. In nineteenth-century Europe and America spa therapies were extremely popular; by the twentieth century they were almost completely ignored. Modern and specialized forms of care replaced each and every indication for traditional balneotherapy, wholly divorcing the spa from its medical origins. In the English-speaking world people now go to mineral springs — or hot tubs — to rest and relax, not to restore their health. Interestingly enough, the recent effort to reintroduce head-out immersion for the medical treatment of circulatory problems has nearly failed; patients refuse to sit in minimal clothing for hours at a time in dreary tubs in the basements of hospitals. Perhaps, as Dr. Harold Conn of Yale University has suggested, if physically attractive nurses of both sexes were recruited to attend bathing patients in pleasant, sunlit surroundings, hospitals, too, might achieve the requisite socialization of the medicinal bath that spas once enjoyed!

Perhaps! However, Western notions of what medicine should be like have changed so radically in the past two centuries that even if hospitals could provide spalike facilities, it is not clear that anyone would take advantage of them. A typical water cure during the eighteenth century lasted twenty-four weeks and required head-out immersion for at least three hours twice a day, three days per week. Who has that kind of time today! Now we expect our medicines to work quickly and to interfere with our lives as little as possible. We are used to the luxury of popping a pill a few times a day or, at worst, getting an injection every so often. Work is now so much more highly valued than rest that it is doubtful any employer or government agency would put up with the lengthy absence of an employee when less time-consuming treatments are available. The fate of medical bathing is a good example of how alterations in the socioeconomic and technological conditions of a society can change the intellectual or perceptual environment of medicine itself.

The recent history of Western medicine is filled with changing perceptions of what medicine is and is not. Spa bathing, bloodletting, the "drawing" of laudable pus, and many herbal preparations succumbed to the new rage for scientific medicine. Maggots used for wound debridement in the years after World War I were dropped once penicillin cleaned up wound care, and surgical and chemical innovations in the 1950s quickly put paid to the use of leeches.

Indeed, leeches were so unlike acceptable medicinal agents in the United States that at least one early proposal to reintroduce them here was totally ignored. In 1943 an American physician named Howard Lilienthal tried to convince his colleagues that the European practice of leeching was far better than simple bed rest for the treatment of thrombophlebitis. The case as he put it was incontrovertible: leeching reduced swelling and pain where the clot was lodged, improved circulation in surrounding tissue, and dissolved the thrombus within a matter of days, thus greatly reducing the length of hospitalization. Nevertheless, Lilienthal's appeal fell on deaf ears. Despite scientific knowledge that leeches not only sucked blood but released anticlotting agents at the bite site — a dual therapy that was difficult to mimic clinically — Americans of the mid-1940s preferred to do without optimal treatment rather than use a leech. Lilienthal and other doctors cognizant of the value of traditional medicines keenly felt the transition to new ways of doing and thinking. "It is surprising that simple drugs should be so extensively prescribed for use in the home, whilst simple physical methods are rarely advocated by the medical men, although they are often of great service," complained one British doctor during the 1930s. "The modern doctor is, I think, 'rather afeared of old wives' remedies,' in case his reputation for science should suffer." Unfortunately, this fearful prejudice is still shared today by many modern physicians who are ignorant of the history and development of their own fields.

We note, however, that doctors have not been alone in rejecting traditional remedies when newer medicines were to be had. Patients, too, have had expectations of what medical treatments should be like. They have objected to maggots crawling in their wounds or leeches sucking up their blood, especially when they could get penicillin or heparin or other efficacious treatments instead. Even something as innocuous as cellophane raised objections from doctors, nurses, and patients when it was first introduced. This clear plastic was simply not what anyone expected a wound dressing to look like, and their negative reaction actually interfered with its use. The fact is that the body cannot be divorced from the mind in treatment.

One can, however, treat the body *through* the mind. When the mind believes that treatment is effective, the body often responds. This placebo effect, as it is called, really can enhance health and the healing process. This is what happens, we suspect, when crippled pilgrims rise and walk after a short dip in spring waters at the religious shrine at Lourdes, France, or when patients report relief from headache after taking a pill that, unknown to them, has no physiological effect. That there must exist an obverse to the placebo effect — it has been called the "nocebo" effect — seems obvious once you think about it: disbelief in or fear of a medical treatment can interfere with or negate the usual physiological benefit.

In its most extreme form, the nocebo effect does not even require actual physical stimulus of the body. This is the case in death by voodoo. If a person truly believes that he can be hexed and someone says she has hexed him, then sheer nerves will make him feel terrible. Instead of interpreting this as fear, he thinks he is ill with the first symptoms of the hex. Believing that there is no cure, he knows it is pointless to eat or drink, and he literally wills himself to death. In experimental situations even well-educated people develop severe headaches from "exposure" to nonexistent electric currents. Research has also shown that the nocebo effect can reverse the body's response to true medical treatment from positive to negative. Patients who believe that they are going to die often do so despite physicians' best efforts.

The presentation of a therapy is therefore as important as its efficacy. And as we stir the melting pot of the world, the lesson becomes more and more urgent. One place where it was taken to heart many years ago was the U.S. Public Health Service's Indian Hospital on the Papago Reservation in Arizona, where physicians have worked side by side with medicine men for decades. "That's hospital policy," said Tim Fleming, the medical director of the hospital in 1976. "If a patient feels there is more to his illness than can be treated by means we provide, and if he or his family want to call in a medicine man, we're glad to cooperate. The hospital is always open to the traditional healers for diagnosis or treatment, day or night. . . . We must walk carefully so that we won't destroy the benefits that they can bring to the Indian patients."

The notion of "culturally sensitive and appropriate health care" — a term that is finally coming into vogue — has been much too long in its genesis. Although it is well documented that most African Americans living in poverty will self-treat and only see qualified physicians as a last resort, almost nothing was known about their folk medicine until a few years ago. According to John Walburn's study of child-care practices, nearly half of the poor African American mothers surveyed clear an infant's nose by placing their mouth over the nostrils and blowing forcefully. Although the practice is effective, Walburn notes that it increases the risk of ear infections. He and his team also found that a quarter of these mothers give infants water before feeding them formula "to flush out the system" and two thirds chew food for their infants. These habits can contribute to malnutrition by dulling the appetite and introducing inappropriate foods into the infant's diet too soon. Physicians cannot evaluate the impact of these practices on a baby's health, however, if they are unsuspected; nor can physicians work with the mothers to correct malnutrition or infection risks without addressing these customs sensitively.

The problems are not limited to any single ethnic group. Latino Americans also self-treat for certain symptoms, relying on home remedies that are mostly unknown or unappreciated by the average American physician. Similarly, although many Asians living in the Americas and Europe still use treatments foreign to conventional Western medicine, such as acupuncture, moxibustion, and herbal remedies, very little was known about the possible benefits and dangers of such therapies until very recently. And in countries disrupted by political violence or civil war, such as Lebanon or Croatia, people regularly resort to home remedies when standard medical supplies disappear. Much more needs to be known about what works and what does not, what interferes with modern medicines and what is complementary to them, before adequate care can be provided in these cases.

We have very far to go. The first nursing journal devoted to culturally appropriate care, *The Journal of Transcultural Nursing*, was founded only in 1989. The physicians' equivalent, *Alternative Therapies in Health and Medicine*, was founded only in 1995. Scientific training has so overwhelmed medical education that most curricula do not even admit that anything else exists. Cultural sensitivity training and concepts of culturally appropriate health care were made available in only 13 of 126 medical schools surveyed in the United States in 1994 and only one of those schools required the course for graduation. Thirty-three additional schools had such courses in the planning stages. As C. K. Lum and S. G. Korenman, the authors of the survey study, concluded, "The results indicate needs for more cultural-sensitivity training and for further studies to determine the most effective type of training for students." Given that sometime in the next few decades more than half the people living in the United States may be of nonwhite ethnic background, this realization is a bit late in coming. That it was overlooked throughout centuries of world domination by European powers is even more distressing. And that we continue to export our scientized, technological medicine to the rest of the world, often in near ignorance of local needs, resources, taboos, and traditions, is inexcusable.

Our point, very simply, is that medicine is no more universal than *Hamlet*. There can be no ultimate, exclusive medicine any more than there is a single best-adapted biological species. The tremendous influence of local environment upon healing in fact requires us to rethink the goals of modern medicine. Adaptation must be the name of the game, for a multicultural world requires many kinds of medicine. We can no longer think in simplistic terms of merely transferring Western medical technology to the rest of the world. We can no longer speak about bringing underdeveloped nations "up" to the "standards" of developed nations. On the contrary, whenever possible, we must rediscover and honor indigenous treatments that are economical as well as effective. And where such treatments do not exist, we must graft Western medicine to the needs of native cultures. In industrialized countries the best care may, indeed, be high-tech, but we must discard the notion that that care be the standard for medicine everywhere in the world.

Paradoxically, recognizing the contextuality of medical care is a first step toward the practice of an optimally evolving medicine. We need not wait for medical treatments to be randomly or accidentally invented in the West. The whole point of this book is to argue that thanks to thousands of years of experimentation, effective treatments already exist in every folk culture around the world. Moreover, experimentation continues in the self-treatment and the use of home remedies that characterize much of alternative medicine today. Without sacrificing the high standards of evidence that modern Western medicine has used to determine effectiveness and safety, we can evaluate these treatments in relation to their cultural environments. Instead of one remedy per disease or injury, we can support many culturally appropriate therapies. And it is not just the Third World that will benefit from this cultural reorientation of medical priorities. Western nations, too, stand to gain in many as yet unforeseen ways. Some indigenous knowledge that has been tested for eons can be, as we have shown, just as useful to us as the latest and most advanced scientific novelties.

Indigenous medical treatments are, in fact, like species of wildlife. The more of them we forfeit to endangerment or extinction for nonmedical reasons, the more we waste of human ingenuity. Some folk medicines have already slipped away. The knowledge gained from experience by Hawaiian *kahunas* has disappeared beyond recall. The last generation of traditional wise men of the Australian aboriginal tribes is dying as we write. The cultural and natural heritage of the peoples of the Brazilian rain forest, driven relentlessly from their jungle homes, vanishes before our very eyes. And we have barely begun to understand what we lose.

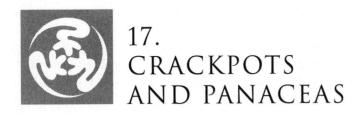

17.
CRACKPOTS
AND PANACEAS

There is nothing people will not do, there is nothing
they have not done, to recover their health and
save their lives. They have submitted to be half
drowned in water, half cooked with gases, to be
buried up to their chins in earth, to be seared with
hot irons like slaves, to be crimped with knives, like
codfish, to have needles thrust into their flesh, and
bonfires kindled on their skin, to swallow all sorts
of abominations, and to pay for all this as if to be
singed and scalded were a costly privilege, as if
blisters were a blessing and leeches were a luxury.

— Oliver Wendell Holmes, M.D., 1891

SOMEWHERE DEEP in our psyches we all want to believe in miracle cures. Every week popular magazines carry articles like the one calling the common weed mullein a "Miracle Drug for Everything from Colds to Bedwetting." Various parts of the plant are said to be good for bleaching and conditioning the hair; treating earaches; curing bedwetting; and relieving coughs, respiratory congestion, and asthma. Take it, you are urged, and you will live longer and prosper.

Every day newspapers nationwide carry full-page ads extolling the putative and equally diverse benefits of vinegar. Vinegar, the ads claim, will soothe sore throats; ward off ear infections; relieve varicose veins, leg cramps, aching muscles, headaches, sunburn, bites, rashes, and itches; stop hiccups and diarrhea; aid digestion and bowel movements; prevent ulcers and urinary tract infections; banish dandruff and pimples; improve skin; remove corns and calluses; "and much, much more . . . ! Just send $12.95 plus $2 shipping to . . ."

And that's not all. You may have taken spicy-hot dishes for mere food, but no more. The cover of the December 19, 1995, *Weekly World News,* a grocery store tabloid, proclaims that "Mustard, Hot Peppers & Horseradish Cure Arthritis, Impotence, Ulcers, Allergies, Acne, Headaches, High Blood Pressure, Warts, Tiredness, Weightloss . . . and much, much more!" Reading further reveals that this "much, much more" includes coughs, deafness, baldness, constipation, flab, stomach ulcers, hemorrhoids, muscle pain, cancer, heart trouble, and colds. Moreover, the tabloid article stresses that these miracle cures are "available in supermarkets everywhere! . . . for just pennies a day," and quotes one (medically unqualified) proponent as saying, "It's not unreasonable to think that they can keep you from ever getting sick again."

Does anyone really believe this kind of nonsense? Does anyone really believe that one remedy can cure all ills? Does anyone really believe, in other words, in panaceas? Absolutely. And doctors have been and are among them. In 1830 an American physician named Marshall Hall thought that bloodletting was almost always called for. "Scarcely a case of acute, or indeed of chronic, disease occurs," he wrote, "in which it does not become necessary to consider the propriety of having recourse to the lancet." Indeed, Hall's book *On the Morbid and Curative Effects of the Loss of Blood* recommended phlebotomy for apoplexy, angina pectoris, dropsy, headaches, palsy, rheumatism, and inflammation of the eyes, bruises, and contusions. So far, perhaps, so good, as we discovered in Chapter 6. But what about the rest of Hall's indications: asthma, vomiting blood, coughs, tuberculosis, diseases of the hip and knee joints, deafness, delirium and lunacy, epilepsy, dizziness, gout, whooping cough, hydrocephalus, inflammation of the lungs, drunkenness, lethargy, lumbago, measles, pleurisy, insomnia, sciatica, shortness of breath, sore throat, and defective perspiration — and (once again) much, much more!

Hall's French contemporary François Broussais similarly prescribed leeches for any and every disease under the sun. Autopsies of hundreds of patients had led him to believe that every disease is characterized by inflammation, particularly of the gastrointestinal tract. He was unaware that immediately following death the intestines release chemicals that stimulate an inflammatory response, causing blood to leak from surrounding tissues and pool in the gut. What Broussais observed in his cadavers, then, was actually an artifact of death, rather than the result of disease. Ignorant of this fact, however, Broussais and his followers often used between ten and fifty leeches per patient, sometimes even before diagnosis, in order to arrest pathological inflammation.

Naturally, the more severe the case, the more leeches were required. One poor woman developed peritonitis, an infection of the abdominal cavity. Broussais, thinking that he understood the nature and causes of her disease from his dissections, applied 250 leeches to the woman's abdomen in less than twenty-four hours in order to suck out the "bad blood." If every one of these leeches had sucked its fill, the woman would have had no blood left at all. As it was, she must have had precious little. She died, but Broussais was not deterred, nor were his followers. One acolyte was so sure that Broussais knew everything about disease and its cure that he infected himself with syphilis, confident that regular leeching at the site of the lesion would quickly cure it. It did not. The syphilis spread throughout the man's body and, full sore, he committed suicide. Undeterred still, Broussais and his true believers went on leeching everyone for everything.

The history of spa therapies reveals a similar strain of fanaticism. The vogue for taking the waters at Bath and other spas is a running theme in the novels of such well-known authors as Jane Austen and Tobias Smollett. Smollett made fun of the people who attended these popular spots and, a doctor himself, of the actual treatments as well. But popular demand fed the medical fad, and physicians took advantage of it. At one time or another during the eighteenth and nineteenth centuries, every disease known to humanity was treated by head-out immersion, wet-sheeting, cold compresses, douching, and other forms of hydrotherapy, as the exuberant and multitudinous use of water, especially cold water, was called. Charles Darwin, who was urged to try all of these things in the 1840s and '50s, noted that even his own doctor was not above a certain faddishness: "It is a sad flaw I cannot but think in my beloved Dr. Gully that he believes in everything."

Nor did such "gullybility" end with the nineteenth century. Around 1900 Dr. P. C. Remondino wrote a book entitled *History of Circumcision from the Earliest Times to the Present* claiming that circumcision could prevent or cure some one hundred different diseases, "including alcoholism, epilepsy, asthma, enuresis, hernia, gout, rectal prolapse, rheumatism, kidney disease, and so forth." Who would have thought that foreskin was so formidable! Or food, for that matter. Virtually the same list of benefits was touted by food faddists such as Charles Kellogg and C. W. Post in the early 1900s. Keeping the bowels properly cleaned out by high-fiber diets, enemas, and exercise, along with electro- and hydrotherapy, could prevent or cure everything from insomnia, lassitude, and chlorosis to abnormal sexual urges, anemia, and cancer. Anyone who has seen the movie *The Road to Wellville* or read T. Coraghessan Boyle's novel of the same name will have gotten an all-too-accurate look at the kind of nonsense that passed as medical salvation at the time. And yet doctors and patients alike flocked to such cures.

Even modern practitioners, yearning as we all do for easy answers, desire panaceas. Erwin Ackerknecht, a medical historian at Yale during the 1950s, stated that during his tenure, his colleagues on the medical faculty seriously believed that the new steroid drug cortisone would cure everything and leave them jobless.

> I will never forget an episode . . . which took place after one of
> the early and obviously overenthusiastic reports on the results

230

of cortisone. Several of my colleagues approached me and said quite seriously and melancholically: "Well, Erwin, you will probably soon be the only man left on this faculty." I could reassure them. But it is almost unbelievable that these experienced men could believe in all earnestness that cortisone could solve all medical problems in the near future.

In the same decade physicians prescribed so much Valium that, according to one estimate, a quarter of all women in the United States were addicted to the drug. If you were depressed, unhappy, dissatisfied with your home life, your work life, or your sex life, you were given Valium. If you had headaches, sleepless nights, anxiety attacks, or nervousness, you were given Valium. It was the midcentury answer to every mental woe. Today we give thanks to Prozac instead. "The history of therapeutics," as Ackerknecht well understood, "reflects all too clearly the human inclination to act according to fashion."

The current popularity of melatonin may be even more instructive. This hormone, which is produced naturally by the body, is sold in the United States not as medicine but as a dietary supplement, placing it outside the jurisdiction of the FDA. At the same time, and without its efficacy ever having been demonstrated in clinical trials, it is being touted by the popular press and by reputable physicians alike as a cure-all for everything from insomnia, breast cancer, and aging, to immune dysfunction. Pandering to panaceas is still medically à la mode.

Therein lies the rub. Every medical procedure, every medical agent, carries a risk. That risk is magnified for folk remedies because they have rarely had to pass the rigorous types of tests demanded of mainstream medical therapies. There are no requirements in folk medicine that records of successes and failures be kept or analyzed. Dangers are often overlooked or, when disaster strikes, ignored or explained away. And even legitimate treatments can be misapplied or extended to symptoms and diseases for which they were not intended and in treating which they can do harm. Thus, although we have carefully documented many

231

ancient and alternative medicines legitimated by modern formal medical practice, we want to focus now on the dangers inherent in thoughtlessly adopting the latest rage in alternative or folk therapies or even in standard medicine.

The hazards are real. For example, mint tea is a favorite home remedy among American Hispanics for treating colicky infants. Unfortunately, one infant died and another became seriously ill recently when their parents gave them such a tea. Unbeknownst to the parents, the tea contained significant amounts of pennyroyal oil, a compound used by other cultures in the past as an abortifacient. Pennyroyal is potentially lethal for any human being and infants are particularly susceptible, often sustaining multiple organ failure. In another recent case, several New Year's Eve revelers at a Los Angeles rock concert stopped breathing, one went into a coma, and thirty-one others became so nauseous and dizzy that they had to be hospitalized after ingesting a supposedly legal herbal stimulant. Natural doesn't always mean safe. Salt water is natural. So are nightshade and hemlock. And they all can be deadly. We therefore need some criteria to differentiate valid medical beliefs from fanciful notions, valid medical experts from crackpots, and useful from harmful concoctions.

To begin with, there are no panaceas and never can be any. This principle was first stated more than two hundred years ago by Enlightenment physicians and philosophers and is generally recognized to be valid today. Every treatment and every drug that has ever claimed to be a panacea has subsequently lost the title. The claims are never borne out by experience.

For one thing, panaceas are impossible for physiological reasons. Drugs work by specific physiological mechanisms that resemble locks and keys. Every cell has a series of "locks" called receptors that mediate communication with the rest of the body and with the environment. Each type of tissue or organ has its own unique set of these receptors — nerves have one type, circulatory system another, reproductive organs a third. Hormones, vitamins, neurotransmitters, and other essential chemicals act like "keys" that can each open one, and only one, of these cellular locks.

Their effects are therefore localized and specific. Drugs generally act by mimicking one of these natural keys and therefore have similarly localized and specific actions. Moreover, these keys are so very different in shape and structure that no equivalent of a skeleton key is possible. Biologically speaking, then, there cannot be a drug that could positively effect every physiological system, and in consequence there can be no panaceas.

Cultural evolution also mediates against the development of panaceas and even against drugs and therapies of very broad medical application. Consider bloodletting and bathing, for example. Both have numerous effects on body systems and represent therapies as close to panaceas as we are likely to find. But the very breadth of their physiological effects has been their own undoing. The development of specialized drugs has allowed physicians to manipulate individual components of these physiological responses more quickly, intensively, and specifically. In the vast majority of cases, the drugs are therefore preferred to the general treatment. Future drugs will have to be even more effective, more specific, and have even fewer side effects to compete with existing ones. The evolutionary trend is therefore toward specialized medicines and away from broadly applicable ones. Even if panaceas could exist physiologically, they would quickly be driven to extinction by the forces directing medical evolution itself.

Unfortunately, panacea pandering is only one characteristic of health-care fraud. Another common criticism of medical crackpots and, by extension, alternative medicines and ancient nostrums is that evidence for their efficacy is anecdotal. The problem with anecdotal evidence is that it is very often selective, retaining only positive results. Consider the following case from the nineteenth century. A man went to a physician for treatment of a kidney complaint. We may assume at this far remove that the problem was most likely kidney stones, a very common problem at the time. Over the next few months the physician repeatedly bled, purged, induced vomiting, scarified, cupped, and generally tried every treatment then in vogue. Finally, and perhaps at his wits' end, the physician applied twelve leeches to the man's anus. Miraculously, he was cured that very day and the physician published his success, claiming he had found a new way to cure kidney complaints!

The physician's mistake was a simple and common one. He confused the temporal correlation between his patient's recovery and his latest treatment as cause and effect. Most likely the patient simply passed the kidney stones on that particular day for reasons totally unassociated with the leeching. But positive correlations are much more memorable than negative ones. We remember the times our horoscope or Chinese fortune cookie fortune comes true; we forget all the times when it does not. That is why the rule in medical science is that a single positive result must be validated by a statistically significant number of additional cases or by direct experiments demonstrating the mechanisms by which the cause exerts its effect. Even more important, all negative results must be compiled and their meanings analyzed. Lamentably, statistically validated medical research originated only in the nineteenth century. Too bad, because many misuses of common therapies might otherwise have been abandoned long before they were. For example, when Charles II of England went into convulsions in February 1685, he was bled, cupped, and scarified; given emetics, purges, and blisters; fed an "emergency forty drops of extract of human skull," and finally forced to swallow a bezoar stone, a concretion from the stomach of a ruminant such as a cow, thought to be an antidote for poison. The king died anyway. Yet every one of these treatments continued to be used for similar symptoms for at least another two hundred years. Too few physicians learned from negative experience. Too few questioned the positive.

Controlled, repeatable observations are also necessary in order to distinguish between effective therapies, which sometimes fail, and noneffective therapies that sometimes "succeed," for instance when recovery is spontaneous and unrelated to treatment. Telling the difference is not easy, as herpetologist Archie Carr has explained in his essay "Bitten by a Fer-de-Lance." Carr was doing field work in Costa Rica when he was bitten by one of these highly poisonous pit vipers. Much to his dismay, he had to wait for transport to the nearest hospital for an entire day. His dilemma was very real. The twenty-four-hour delay in treatment posed a great risk, since by the time he reached the hospital most antivenin treatments available there would no longer be able to prevent death. Should he opt for the equally risky emergency serum in his own kit that might also prove fatal? Carr held off and, finding himself still alive after some hours, he began to believe that perhaps the snake had not actually injected poison with the bite.

For unknown reasons, the fer-de-lance sometimes conserves its venom. And when Carr finally made it to the hospital he learned that this had been the case. But his experience set him to thinking about the many local snake-bite "cures" he had been told of during his long hours of worry. Next time you are bitten, he was told, kill the snake, mash up the brain, and smear it into the wound. It will soak up the poison. Alternatively, rub kerosene into the bite; chew tobacco; drink coffee. Do any of these folk remedies work? Probably not, but if antivenin shots are unavailable, a person faced with imminent death will try anything. "And if the incidence of aborted bites is high enough," notes Carr, "the cure would be bound to take hold as part of the folk medicine of the country. If generations keep getting 40 percent recovery from snake brains, kerosene, and chewing tobacco, they have to be unnaturally skeptical not to stick to these treatments. Modern medicine has few specifics that cure at such a rate."

The critical point is that, in many cases, anything works no better than nothing. Most diseases have a limited course, remissions occur unexpectedly in the presence of treatment, and spontaneous cures occur in its absence. Unless we know how frequent the natural reversal of disease is likely to be, we cannot evaluate the efficacy of a treatment. Individual cases and even uncontrolled collections of statistics won't suffice because it is the *change* in the success rate, and not the absolute percentage or number of successes, that counts.

In modern medicine, therefore, any correlation, whether between leeching and relief from kidney stones or between mashed snake brains and snake-bite survival, is spurious until proven otherwise. It would be a mistake, however, to discard all unique observations or anecdotal reports out of hand. Jenner, remember, began his researches on the protective actions of cowpox based on a single anecdote he heard as a teenager from a milkmaid. Withering began his investigations of foxglove based on an observation of a single case. So did the inventors of cellophane bandages. Single observations and anecdotal reports are crucial spurs to medical progress. They are the initial clues to something unexpected and exciting, the often serendipitous events that change the course of an investigation. But we must always remember that such clues can be red herrings, unique anomalies, unreproducible flukes of happenstance, too. Scientific research is more than just finding something new. It is a *process* involving observation, validation, and verification, a journey that, as in the old Chinese saying about all journeys, begins with a single step. To be successful, one must take both the first step *and* the journey it presages.

Many crackpots confuse the first step with the entire trip. Others fall prey to a different sort of confusion. They think that running all over the place is the same as purposeful travel. Their philosophy seems to be: do everything to everybody and something will emerge. It is true that to take the research journey, one must enlarge the number of patients treated and compare their progress with others who receive different therapies. One must also use trial and error to determine the range of symptoms for which the new treatment may be valid, as Withering did with digitalis. But Withering's research was carefully directed and limited. Having guessed at the mechanism by which digitalis worked, he tested his drug on diseases that all had water retention or circulatory problems as common symptoms. The key at this stage of the research journey is to map carefully the newfound field and determine its boundaries, not to run helter-skelter all over creation.

What all panaceas have in common is just this helter-skelter application of a single treatment to the widest possible range of unrelated conditions. Having taken one successful step, hucksters — whether medically accredited or not — run amuck, performing experiments uncritically on every known disease. Invariably, the "results" are touted to an ignorant public before the data are in and without comparison to other, standard treatments. Worse, the basic fundamentals of physiology, pharmacology, or other medical fields are overlooked. For example, we know enough to say that a medicine that treats sore throats is unlikely to have an appreciable effect on cancer, or that a remedy for heart disease is unlikely to benefit a person suffering from psoriasis. And yet just such silly claims are made daily for panaceas, though the very nature of the claims should make us suspicious.

A woman named Bonnee Hendricks Hoy provides an illustrative case. Diagnosed by a legitimate physician as having cervical cancer in 1983, she was told she had a 90 percent probability of complete remission if she had an immediate hysterectomy. Hoy was convinced by some nutritionists, however, to forgo surgery in favor of a macrobiotic diet based entirely on vegetables and designed to correct the "imbalances" in her body that had supposedly allowed the cancer to manifest itself. The fact that most cervical cancers are caused by chronic papilloma virus infections was ignored. Like Broussais, who believed that all disease was caused by gastrointestinal inflammation, these nutritionists believed that all diseases stem from improper nutrition. After six months on her new diet, these medically untrained "healers" proclaimed Hoy 70 percent cured. Two months later she died.

Whatever (questionable) nutritional benefits macrobiotic diets may confer on some people, there is no medical evidence and no reason to believe that they can have any effect whatever on an existing cancer. Reputable physicians may use nutrition as part of cancer therapy, as an adjunct to surgery, chemotherapy, or radiation, but never as a treatment by itself. The macrobiotic nutritionists had no business experimenting on a person who had every reason to believe she would be cured by the standard medical procedures. In a rational world, or one in which our standards of education were higher, she would have known not to believe them.

Another common excess indulged in by crackpots is the belief that if a small amount of something is good, more is better.

According to the physician and historian Guido Majno, this is exactly where many practitioners in ancient and medieval times went wrong with laudable pus. They thought that if a little pus was good, lots of it was even better. Bloodletting followed the same path, ushering in an era of "sanguinary" physicians and "heroic medicine" that often ended in death. A classic example involves George Washington, who as an old man developed a severe sore throat, perhaps of streptococcal origin. His physician, a Dr. Craik, bled him to faintness four times in two days, until Washington begged him not to do so again. By then it is likely that Washington had lost two quarts or more of blood. He died within hours of his last bleeding, and Craik conceded afterward that perhaps he had let too much blood. But the admission came too late.

A more recent example concerns one Ruth Conrad, who visited a naturopath, a medically unaccredited person who specializes in natural remedies, for treatment of arthritis. In addition to treating the arthritis, the naturopath also "diagnosed" a small bump on Conrad's nose as being cancerous and gave her some black ointment to put on it. The ointment burned terribly when Conrad applied it, so she called the naturopath on the telephone to complain. He told her that the burning proved she really had cancer and she should keep using the remedy until the burning stopped. Conrad ended up in the hospital five days later. And no one ever found out whether she really had had a cancerous lesion, because she suffered such terrible chemical burns from the ointment that seventeen plastic surgeries were required to rebuild her nose. The ointment the naturopath had given her contained zinc chloride, sometimes used in very weak dilutions in human and animal medicines as an antiseptic or astringent, but also used at higher concentrations to etch metal and brown steel. The naturopath had clearly provided Conrad with a very potent mixture to take care of a very serious problem. In this instance, both the "healer" and the patient were remiss in not knowing when too much was too much.

Dr. Stephen Barret, an expert on quackery, and FDA officials note that medical crackpots and charlatans have several other relatively common traits. First, they tend to have questionable medical credentials. The National Council Against Health Fraud says that people can easily obtain phony certification as cancer researchers or nutritionists through the mail from institutions such as Bernadian University and the Nutritionists Institute of America. One health-care fraud investigator even got his dog certified by the American Association of Nutrition and Dietary Consultants! Experts caution consumers to look for health-care providers who have legitimate degrees from well-known and established universities.

Second, quacks almost always claim to be able to cure what standard medicines cannot. Note that even the best of the treatments we have described in this book, such as honey and head-out immersion, are generally used only as last resorts by modern physicians. Only a handful of alternative and folk therapies actually perform better than standard medicines. The most successful folk treatments are *sources* for modern medicines, not miracle cures. Any treatment that is espoused as a panacea is immediately suspect.

Third, to "prove" their seductive claims, frauds usually cite pop-medicine books, unpublished studies, anecdotal evidence, satisfied customers, or their own experience rather than papers published in major medical journals. This is a sure tip-off that the treatment has not been validated. When challenged about the lack of validation, the fraud will most often claim that orthodox doctors are either too close-minded to consider the treatment or too worried that it will put them out of business. Some frauds even use paranoid language about how the medical profession is "out to get them." More likely, doctors already know of studies that have proven these treatments inefficacious, even downright dangerous. This is certainly the case for some of the most recent fraudulent medical nostrums: laetrile, DMSO (dimethyl sulfoxide), chelation therapy, and many nutritional supplements.

Unavailable in the United States, Canada, or Europe, laetrile is a compound that is touted in some places, such as Mexico, as a cure-all for cancers. Laboratory studies have found, however, that it has no effect on cancer whatsoever. People exchanging proven therapies for laetrile are throwing away their best chance at life. DMSO is a well-known and widely used chemical solvent that is supposed to cure arthritis. While it may have some antiinflammatory activity, it has no established effects on arthritic disease. What it does have is the ability to pass through otherwise impermeable skin, carrying chemical toxins piggyback. Physicians consider it a dangerous substance. As a cure for atherosclerosis, chelation therapy involves the extraction of various key minerals, such as calcium and iron, from the bloodstream, presumably to prevent hardening of the arteries. Again there are no known benefits from this form of treatment, and numerous cases of severe illness and death are on record. People who toy with these and many other alternatives risk their health and their lives.

For these reasons, particular care must be exercised by people with diseases that are essentially incurable using standard medical therapies, such as AIDS, various forms of cancer, arthritis, multiple sclerosis, and Crohn's disease. They owe it to themselves to learn as much about their disease and its treatment as they possibly can, for health-care frauds are easiest to perpetrate on people who are the most desperate and the least educated about medicine. As one woman with arthritis recently said, "You get to a point where you're willing to try almost anything." That is exactly what charlatans want to hear.

But what of alternative or ethnic treatments offered by well-established physicians? What do you do if Dr. Mehmet Oz of Columbia-Presbyterian Hospital in New York wants to have healer Julie Motz stand over you and funnel what the Chinese call *qi-gong* — some sort of healing energy that no one can prove exists — into your body during your cardiac bypass operation? What do you say to Dr. Deepak Chopra when he urges you to adopt Ayurvedic eating habits in conjunction with his more standard prescription to exercise more to control stress-related diseases, or to Dr. Dean Ornish when he urges you to meditate or practice yoga to lower your risk of heart attack? How can the average person evaluate these sorts of suggestions?

240

Very simply, we should ask of alternative treatments the same proofs of efficacy and safety that we demand of standard medical care. Note that Oz, Chopra, Ornish, and other reputable physicians advocating non-Western medical approaches limit them to essentially no-risk adjunctive therapies. If Ayurvedic medicine or yoga works for you, that's great. If not, no harm will be done. These doctors do not eliminate the use of standard medicines. They promise no miracles and make no sweeping claims. If you ask them, you will learn that they are engaged in properly controlled studies to find out whether these treatments really work and, if so, how. They have not already decided, as medical shysters have, that these new therapies are miraculous breakthroughs. As Ornish says, "There is great value in almost any of these traditions, but each in limited circumstances. Not everything works for everybody."

The problem is, few alternative or folk treatments are as risk-free as *qi-gong*. They may require giving up standard medicines, be inherently dangerous, or simply lack validation. In the preliminary evaluation of these treatments we suggest that an additional biorational criterion may come in handy. Those therapies most likely to be of value are ones that have very long histories of continuous use in many different cultures. The phenomena of long-term survival and convergence in the evolution of medicine strongly suggest that something efficacious and adaptive is at the heart of a therapy. Every one of the treatments discussed in this book satisfies this requirement. This evolutionary criterion also allows us to avoid fads and fashions. To participate in the latest alternative medical craze is to become a human guinea pig. Anyone who does so should understand the risks.

Even the criterion of long-term use, however, requires a caveat. Every culture has its crackpots and panaceas and some survive for eons. Just because a custom is widespread and long-standing does not *guarantee* medical validity. In his encounter with native antidotes to snake poisoning, Archie Carr provided illustration of the sort of false correlation between treatment and outcome that can keep nonefficacious practices alive. Efficacy must be real, if we are to take a folk medicine seriously. For this reason, the same criteria we use to distinguish crackpot from real medicine in our own culture should guide us in distinguishing between those indigenous beliefs and practices we may legitimately press other peoples to relinquish and those we ought to respect for their medical efficacy and cultural fit. No one ought to deny Ethiopians access to chloroquine in the treatment of porphyria cutanea tarda, even though that drug does not provide optimal medicine. By the same token, no one ought to argue that native peoples in Africa or elsewhere may rightly resist medical treatment when that resistance puts themselves — and the rest of the world — at risk. In Uganda and Zaire, for example, where promiscuity is common, circumcision is rare, use of condoms is considered "unmanly," and high-tech drugs are virtually nonexistent, men and their sexual partners have essentially no protection against the rampant spread of STDs and AIDS. Western medicine has an obligation to honor culturally acceptable *efficacious* forms of treatment. It also has an obligation to urge change where indigenous treatments are clearly ineffective or nonexistent. To do otherwise is to condone fraudulent medicine.

Consider a case in point: smallpox vaccination. Cultural resistance to vaccination has, as we have seen, a long past, including European resistance to the Asian practice and American Indian resistance to European. Ed Regis, a medical writer, notes that such resistance continued in various parts of the world well into this century:

> During the 1960's, when doctors from the World Health Organization set out to eradicate smallpox, they were faced with indigenous beliefs in the local smallpox gods. In India it was the goddess Shitala; in Africa it was the god Shapona; in the New World — in Brazil and some other parts of Latin America — it was the god Omolou. Believers claimed that vaccinating people would elicit the wrath of the smallpox gods, causing unbridled outbreaks of the disease.

Despite indigenous fears, the WHO pressed forward in its campaign to deliver smallpox vaccination worldwide. Not to have done so would have been gross negligence, for mass vaccination not only saved millions of lives throughout Africa, Asia, and Latin America, it also protected people around the world from the scourge. A disease with no reservoir, no unprotected host population, cannot survive. Because of the WHO's vaccination efforts, no case of smallpox has been documented anywhere in the world for more than twenty years. The disease has been officially eradicated.

Respect for other medical cultures cannot, therefore, include thoughtless acceptance of any or all practices and beliefs. We are all put at medical risk or economic expense when treatable conditions are left untreated to satisfy local customs. It would be a mistake to condone crackpot medicine, no matter where we find it. The challenge lies in reconciling the need for efficacious medicine with the need for a culturally sensitive medicine; it lies in distinguishing clearly between good and bogus treatments, not only within Western culture but among medical cultures the world over. The fact is, as medicine evolves worldwide, it will slowly but surely drive inefficacious treatments to extinction. Many old wives' tales and alternative therapies will not survive the competition.

With respect to our own medical culture and its ongoing evolution, our point is simple. Old is not necessarily good. Natural is not necessarily better. Folk remedies used in technologically undeveloped countries are not necessarily worth investigating for use in the West. In the highly sophisticated niche created by the industrial world, ancient and alternative medicines are not necessarily more suitable than standard practice. Sometimes they may be, as the many folk remedies and old wives' tales in this book suggest. In general, however, the medicines developed and used in technologically advanced societies are the best any culture has found. We need to measure alternative therapies against this current standard before we adopt them. In no instance should our own medical past or foreign indigenous practice in the present be a direct guide to modern Western practice.

No reasonable person would suggest that we in the West return to the days of bloodletting, poultices, patent medicines, and laudable pus. There is no reason to eat clay from the brickyard instead of vitamin supplements or Kaopectate, and there are many reasons not to. Saliva and urine might save lives in an emergency, but they are no substitutes for the sterilized, purified components we have isolated from them. Rather, the object in looking to the past or to other medical cultures for insight into present biomedical problems is to identify the useful elements that lie buried amid the outmoded, unsound, even detrimental trappings of other medicines and use them to stimulate our own medicine to ever greater achievement. It takes skepticism and analysis to tease what is valuable out of the dross of history and anthropology. Doing this well and doing it properly is an essential guard against the dangers of crackpots and panaceas.

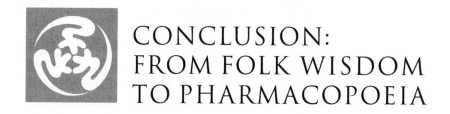

CONCLUSION:
FROM FOLK WISDOM
TO PHARMACOPOEIA

Much profit can be obtained by renewing old studies,
using a somewhat different approach. I think in
the future there will be much revitalization of old
knowledge, but it must be revitalized.

— Chandler M. Brooks, Ph.D., 1966

WHAT, FINALLY, of old wives' tales in the future? The path from folk wisdom to professional acceptance has never been an easy one. Jenner found the path to vaccination rocky, to say the least. Withering encountered severe resistance to the use of digitalis. Disbelief also met the medical innovators who reintroduced honey and sugar pastes, the supporters of head-out immersion therapies, the developers of cellophane and other plastic bandages, and all the other mavericks we have described.

Resistance to innovation is an inescapable part of evolutionary competition. No one gives up their cherished beliefs or habitual modes of action without a fight. There is no reason, therefore, to expect the incorporation of folk therapies into mainstream medicine to be easy or simple in the future. Nor should this process be too easy. Many home remedies deserve to go extinct. The critical problem is this: some alternatives do deserve to be incorporated into standard medical practice but, in the current system, cannot be. Two contemporary cases, one involving light therapies and the other a chemical called DNCB, illustrate the kinds of

245

barriers that exist. The specific nature of the barriers these treatments face in turn suggests potential solutions.

Light therapies have been known for hundreds, if not thousands, of years. One of their most common modern uses is to treat seasonal affective disorder (SAD), a form of depression associated with the long, dark winter months in northern regions of the world and in places with persistent cloudy, rainy weather. One effective treatment for SAD is to expose its sufferers to very bright lights for an hour or more every day. Light treatment for SAD has been under study for decades and has been in fairly general use for many years. Light therapies are also commonly used to treat disturbed sleep patterns associated with night-shift work and overseas travel. While physicians often charge for the use of facilities and equipment that deliver light therapies, no one has ever claimed economic rights to control the dispensing of such therapies by physicians.

The medical and research communities were therefore shocked in 1994 when Harvard University investigators filed patents covering most of the therapeutic uses of light. A controversy quickly developed that has focused on two aspects of the patent claims. First, many researchers and physicians contend that most of the information used to support the Harvard patent claims has been in the public domain for a considerable period of time. According to patent law, anything that is general knowledge or, in patent lingo, "obvious" to practitioners in the field cannot be patented. This provision causes clear-cut problems for almost any form of folk medicine since all such medicines are, by their very nature, publicly known. Unless a medical researcher discovers some new active ingredient that is previously unknown to both lay and professional practitioners, most folk medicines by themselves cannot be patented.

The second issue concerns economics. The Harvard researchers claim that if patent rights cannot be secured for light therapies, then it will be impossible to commercialize them. The commercial considerations are not simply a matter of greed. Medical therapies cannot be marketed or distributed in the United

States or in most other countries without the approval of the Food and Drug Administration or an equivalent regulatory body. The FDA-mandated tests for efficacy and safety require large-scale clinical trials that often cost on the order of $10 to $20 million. This is only a small part of the total cost of drug development. Current estimates of the cost from the initial discovery or observation to the production of a marketable medical product are $250 million. The Harvard investigators argue quite plausibly that no commercial enterprise is likely to invest tens or hundreds or millions of dollars to develop a light therapy and push it through the FDA approval process without some assurance that their investment is protected. That is the purpose of a patent. It secures the holder a guaranteed period of seventeen to twenty years (depending on the country in which it is issued) during which the holder has exclusive rights to manufacture and market the therapy. This grace period allows the patent holder to recoup his or her substantial investment. Patentability therefore facilitates marketability.

Once again the implications for folk medicines are manifest. The critical issue is marketability. Any physician can put honey on a wound without FDA approval because she is administering a food agent exempt from medical regulations. She may also prescribe any other unregulated agent therapeutically. No individual or organization may, however, *market* honey or anything else as a therapeutic agent without FDA approval, since the FDA regulates all claims of medical safety and efficacy *in the marketplace*. To avoid such regulation, many herbal remedies are therefore sold as nutritional supplements rather than medicines and may not make any medical claims in their packaging or advertising.

In order for an agent to become a part of the standard pharmacopoeia, it must be marketed as a medicine and acquire FDA approval. The costs of carrying out the tests to acquire this approval exist whether the treatment is patentable or not. Thus one of the safeguards of modern medicine — controlled scientific testing — presents an economic hurdle many folk remedies cannot surmount. Who is going to invest the many millions of dollars necessary to bring the treatment to the medical market if no patent is possible and if any pharmaceutical company, distributor, or practitioner can then provide the same treatment without having invested a cent in its development?

The problems are further exacerbated by the widespread availability and inordinate cheapness of the ingredients of most folk remedies. Nearly everyone has access to honey, sugar, cellophane, and many of the other folk medicines we have described. This accessibility also plagues dinitrochlorobenzene, or DNCB, a chemical that is currently being studied for its enhancement of immune-system activity. DNCB is best known to the public as photographic developer. Photographers learned decades ago not to put their hands in developer; if they did, they got a terrible rash that turned the affected skin red, swollen, and itchy. Immunologists found that the developer stimulates an allergic response that turns up immune-system activity in the entire body. DNCB was therefore tried, with some success during the 1970s, as an adjunct therapy for people whose immune systems were damaged by cancer chemotherapy. Several studies have suggested that it promotes tumor regression.

When AIDS arrived on the scene during the 1980s, many people infected with HIV quickly gave up on standard medical approaches, since none of the drugs prescribed by mainstream researchers seemed to have much effect on the progress of the disease. Groups such as Act Up, Gay Men's Health Crisis centers, and many local organizations began collecting information on any therapy, whatever its origin, that might be medically beneficial. These have included nutritional supplements, Asian herbs, and Hindu therapies, as well as standard pharmaceuticals. Among the drugs identified in this process was DNCB. Since AIDS is characterized by the slow decay of the immune system, and DNCB stimulates immune function, controlled exposure to DNCB was proposed as a possible way to restore the immune system.

Community-sponsored clinical trials of DNCB run by Raphael Stricker and B. F. Elswood in San Francisco have, in fact, shown that when the drug is swabbed regularly on a small patch of skin, it appears to slow the progress of AIDS during its early stages. The problem is that DNCB is too inexpensive to be of any interest to pharmaceutical companies. The new protease inhibitors and classical therapies for HIV treatment, such as AZT or multidrug regimens, are estimated to cost $8,000 to $15,000 per year per patient and require medical supervision. There is lots of money to be made. In contrast, a year of DNCB treatment costs $20 and can be self-administered by the patient. In comparison with standard anti-HIV therapies, there is simply no profit in DNCB, which, in any case, is unpatentable. Any company attempting to bring the treatment to market will need FDA approval but will not be able to protect its investment. Groups attempting to drum up interest in this therapy have therefore been uniformly rebuffed by the pharmaceutical industry.

Our point here is not to argue that DNCB is better than other AIDS treatments — large-scale clinical trials such as the FDA would require have never been run — but rather to emphasize that the issues determining its long-term evaluation depend only partially on its medical benefits. Even if DNCB were substantially better than existing treatments, its pharmaceutical potential would still be evaluated by the industry mainly on its *marketability*. This is a critical factor in the dissemination of *all* new therapies, both mainstream and alternative. Unless someone can figure out how to allow business to benefit from the use of DNCB — and by extrapolation, honey, cellophane, and other efficacious folk medicines — they have little chance of surviving outside of experimental settings. They cannot be marketed as pharmaceutical agents despite their medical benefits. Efficacy is not, and has never been, enough.

How then can we expect old wives' tales to survive modern competition with formalized medical care? Given the current situation in industrialized nations, there appear to be only five basic ways in which folk medicines can survive in the modern medical market: first, by providing patentable therapeutic agents or processes that can be developed commercially in the accepted manner; second, by filling a niche that standard therapies cannot address;

third, by providing cost benefits sufficiently large that savings, rather than profits, drive their adoption; fourth, by surviving as FDA-unapproved alternatives to standard medicine; and fifth, by generating enough public support that demand drives their supply.

The first and perhaps most common way folk remedies have survived in modern medicine is by providing new and patentable therapeutic substances. We have already discussed the fact that pharmaceutical and biotechnology companies have isolated and developed a wide range of drugs from urine, saliva, leeches, and other sources. In these instances, folk wisdom yielded up complex therapies that harbored many active ingredients unknown to the public and science alike. Novel agents such as histatins, growth factors, muramyl dipeptide, urokinase, hirudin, and hementin are patentable and have sufficiently large markets that companies profit by developing them. The most controversial aspect of this development process is whether drugs or therapies based on folk wisdom *should* be patentable and, if so, who should control the patent rights.

These issues loom ever larger as more and more insights are gleaned from indigenous cultures in South America, Africa, Asia, and the South Pacific. There is increasing demand worldwide that the appropriate ethnic groups, or the countries in which they reside, be given some portion of the proceeds of any patentable therapy that results from their folk medicines. Issues of international and intellectual property rights in such transactions will undoubtedly take many years to sort out. One that has gotten too little attention in these discussions is the possibility that money may not always be the culturally appropriate payment for such rights. We may want to think about what services we can provide to non-Western cultures that benefit them in ways equivalent, but not identical, to the ways in which we benefit. For example, a rain-forest tribe that provides us with a new cancer agent might benefit most by having the pharmaceutical company that develops the drug buy up and donate to them as a preserve their home lands. That way the natural and cultural environments that provided the medical intuition in the first place will continue to exist and may provide other drug sources.

The second way in which folk medicines can reinvigorate modern medicine is to fill niches that current therapies cannot. Right now maggots and leeches perform functions that no surgeon and no drug can perform. Businesses such as Roy Sawyer's Biopharm, which supplies leeches worldwide, can afford to provide these therapeutic agents to hospitals because there are no direct medical competitors. Similarly, honey and sugar preparations are used when antibiotics, antiseptics, and surgery fail. They are courts of last resort. Even Sawyer, who profits from his leech farm, expects, someday, to put the farm out of business. His true goal is "to isolate the useful chemicals from their [leeches'] saliva and reproduce them in the laboratory for pharmaceutical use." Live leeches are just a stopgap.

Economics can create niches as well. In some countries, such as India and parts of Africa, cellophane is still a viable alternative to expensive bandaging materials. One can imagine disasters or wars in which these various treatments would all become more prevalent, even in the best hospitals. Nevertheless, there are limitations on the likelihood of folk wisdom being used in preference to modern medicines in the West. In almost all the cases that we have documented, the operative factor is that the medical condition is serious, possibly fatal, and modern medicines are absolutely not available or have failed. Except in disaster scenarios, alternative medicines will survive in industrialized nations only where modern medicines have not yet done better. Our cultural preferences encourage the development, not of ancient or alternative medicines, but rather of their replacements, as must be clear from the continued efforts of physicians over a hundred years ago and again today to design a mechanical leech. Cultural competition is tough on ancient remedies. By the same token, therapies that have survived millennia of use and still outperform the best that modern medicine can invent have got to be damn good!

The real question is how one gets treatments like honey or sugar pastes, light therapies, perhaps DNCB, and other possibly highly effective but unpatentable agents into general use. Doctors can try anything in emergencies. They cannot sell these catch-as-catch-can experiments to the public. However, many nonpatentable agents exist as part of natural healing regimens, some of which would undoubtedly also be candidates for widespread use but for their nonmarketability. Here a third possibility needs to be considered. Rather than focusing on profit potential, which for agents like honey and DNCB is generally very small, we suggest that the focus be placed on the potential for cost *savings*.

The economics of medical care are very complex, involving not only pharmaceutical and biotechnology companies but physicians and patients, hospitals, insurers, and state and federal governments. If there is both a standard pharmaceutical treatment and an alternative folk medicine for a given medical problem, and one can show that the alternative medicine is not only equally efficacious but substantially less expensive, then patients, hospitals, and insurers, including the government, stand to benefit. At least one such treatment already exists. Honey and sugar pastes not only cure ulcers and infected burns that standard therapies cannot, they also speed healing, cut the number of hospital visits dramatically, and decrease the need for plastic surgery. DNCB may represent another possibility for the treatment of AIDS, if not in industrialized countries, certainly in impoverished ones. Assuming that the Harvard light therapy patent applications will not be granted, then light therapy also qualifies, since it is much less expensive to deliver than psychiatric or drug therapies for depression. The question is how to capitalize on these potential savings.

Here we make a novel suggestion. Since hospitals, medical insurers, and the government are the institutions that stand to benefit most from the cost savings, we suggest that they form consortia to underwrite the development, testing, and dissemination of cost-effective nonpatentable therapies (NPTs). We imagine such NPT consortia being modeled on the Underwriters Laboratory, which was established by the home insurance industry to set standards for electrical appliances and thereby prevent costly electrical disasters. In this case, the goal would be to provide high-quality care at the lowest possible price.

We suggest very demanding criteria for the development of NPTs. Obviously, they must be nonpatentable according to the criteria laid down by patent examiners. Most important, they should have the potential for treating diseases that are currently untreatable with standard medical therapies or should allow substantial clinical savings in comparison with existing therapies. The medical insurance consortia, aided by existing government institutions such as the Alternative Medicine Program of the National Institutes of Health, would then fund the research and development necessary for these NPTs to satisfy criteria for FDA approval. If the FDA approves an alternative therapy that lowers medical costs sufficiently, insurers can more than recoup their investment by mandating preferential use of these therapies for insured patients. The development and production of NPTs could be undertaken as a public service by public universities having appropriate research and medical facilities. Since the NPTs would be supplied to the medical community at cost, the benefit to the universities would lie in large-scale, long-term funding and the prestige of training large numbers of investigators and clinicians. We suspect that as health-care costs continue to climb, we may have no choice but to move in this direction.

In the meantime, it is clear that alternative medicines will continue to survive, as they have throughout all of modern medical history, in a fourth way, outside of standard medical care and the FDA-approval process. While the FDA determines what can be sold or prescribed as medicine, it has no control over things that are not sold for medical use. Thus anyone can buy honey and sugar, cellophane, ginseng, aloe vera, and hundreds of other folk remedies without regulation.

The danger here, however, is that folk remedies, as we have stressed, can be and often are dangerous when used by the uninitiated. In traditional cultures wise women, shamans, witch doctors, and natural healers learn their craft over a lifetime. They learn when to pick their plants, because if harvested at the wrong time of year or in the wrong place, plants may be deadly instead of restorative. They learn how to prepare their materials and in what amounts, because if prepared improperly the materials may cause illness instead of cure, poison instead of soothe. This sort of understanding does not come packaged with folk remedies bought at health-food stores or delivered by neighborhood naturopaths. Thus this fourth way of preserving nontraditional medical wisdom is not one we favor. Self-treatment has too many risks. We would prefer to see the wisdom of the past dispensed by experts who understand their job. We would like even better to have that wisdom tested and, if it is adequate, incorporated into the standard medical corpus in the ways we have illustrated in this book.

The fifth and final way in which alternative medicines can survive in the modern world is to become sufficiently popular that public demand results in their being supplied by mainstream health-care providers even without full-scale medical testing or approval. To some extent this is already happening. With 60 to 80 percent of the world still using traditional medical therapies — or what physicians in industrialized countries call complementary or alternative medicines — and with the widespread travel and immigration that characterize our modern world, the geographical and cultural insulation of Western medicine has broken down. Individuals unhappy with modern medical care for reasons of cost, quality, or effectiveness are increasingly turning toward alternative medicines, now within easy reach.

In many cases they do so with their doctors' blessings. More and more private practitioners are also beginning to experiment with alternatives. Among them is Dr. Brian Berman, who found himself unable to alleviate the painful facial paralysis due to trigeminal neuralgia in one of his patients. Out of frustration, Berman turned to a homeopathic (or incredibly diluted) preparation of belladonna and causticum. While homeopathy has no scientific basis, Berman and his patient claim the alternative treatment worked, and as far as they are concerned, that's all that matters. Dr. Nancy Dickey, chair of the board of directors of the

American Medical Association, summed up this new attitude by saying, "If I had a patient who said, 'I quit using codeine since I started doing acupuncture,' I'd say, 'Terrific.'" The attitude "do what works for your patient" is becoming more and more common.

It is so common, in fact, that forty-one states now require medical insurers to cover chiropractic therapy, six require insurers to cover acupuncture, and one, Washington State, requires insurers to cover alternative medicines in general. At the same time, some health maintenance organizations (HMOs) around the country have decided on their own initiative to pay for chiropractic treatments, acupuncture, massage therapy, yoga, and certain herbal remedies. Medical industry analysts say the HMOs have found that people who utilize such alternatives tend to be healthier than the general run-of-the-mill patient and so cost the HMO less. In other words, it is profitable to attract the business of alternative medicine enthusiasts, whether the therapies they receive are truly effective or not.

There are, however, real dangers in medical change driven by popular demand. We have already seen that physicians feel the same pressures for miracle cures and panaceas that the rest of us do. As David L. Gollaher of the California Health Care Institute has noted, it is sometimes very difficult to determine who leads and who follows in the dance that becomes a medical fad:

> From their residencies onward, most doctors discover that pressure to conform to what is considered standard within the local medical community is irresistible. In turn, these practice standards, imbued as they are with medical authority, shape patients' preferences. For patients normally presume that what doctors accept as medical policy is also the best thing to do. . . . The doctor-patient relationship contains a built-in mechanism of mutual reinforcement, encouraging both parties to follow the pack. With the passage of time some practices harden within medical and popular culture alike so it becomes impossible to sort out how much demand for a

procedure should be attributed to physicians and how much
to patients.

Doctors are in business, and one of the rules of all successful
businesses is that the customer is always right. If providing patients
with treatments that keep them coming back is necessary to keep
the shingle hanging on the door, many physicians will do so. By
allowing popular demand to push the direction of medical care,
there is a real risk that we will encounter new fads as outrageous as
those that led at various times to indiscriminate bloodletting and
compulsory leeching of every patient, head-out immersion for
every chronic symptom, tonsillectomy for every sore throat, ster-
oids and antibiotics for every ache and fever.

The challenges of finding, evaluating, and marketing efficacious folk remedies and alternative therapies require Western physicians and medical consumers to rethink the nature of medical
research. It is human nature to want to stay within the comfortable
light of current knowledge. Similarly, it is human nature to reject
what does not fit our preconceptions. For this reason, every discovery is a surprise. We must court surprises by learning where
they are most likely to be hidden. We must learn to admit that
where long-standing medical problems exist, there are no experts,
no superior sources of knowledge. If the experts had the answers,
then the problems would not persist. Learning to learn from non-
professional venues thus becomes as important to the medical
sciences as mastering medical practice or technique.

Medical researchers and health-care providers must therefore open their eyes to the huge debt that medicine owes to insightful laypeople, past and present, and balance the need for
learned skepticism with an open mind. Dr. Marlys Witte and phi-
losopher Ann Kerwin of the University of Arizona Medical School
teach their students one way of doing this in their "Curriculum on
Medical Ignorance." There are four basic kinds of ignorance, according to Witte and Kerwin: things we think we know but really
don't (ignorance masquerading as knowledge); things we know
we don't know (overt ignorance); things we don't know we don't

know (hidden ignorance); and things we don't know we do know (knowledge masquerading as ignorance).

Our awareness of these kinds of ignorance has a direct hand in the task of finding and evaluating medical insights in unlikely places. Folk traditions and the idiosyncratic experiments of laypeople are two of the best sources of information we don't know we do know and sometimes reveal the holes in what we thought we knew, as well. Learning to recognize ignorance enables us to transform it into questions that may yield new answers to outstanding medical problems. This ability is as critical to medical progress as is all the expert knowledge in the world, for it will help the practitioner listen to the tales of an old wise woman, an attending nurse, or a sick patient with well-formulated problems in mind and a discriminating ear. William Withering, Edward Jenner, and William Baer possessed this talent and so do David Werner, Martín, and the other members of Project Projimo today. It is a talent worth cultivating.

Challenging medical ignorance with the insights of folk remedies and alternative therapies also requires a new kind of medical professional who can bridge cultures. Companies such as Shaman Pharmaceuticals and other biotechnology groups that are actively pursuing ethnopharmacological leads need people prepared adequately and concurrently in medicine, botany or pharmaceutical research, anthropology or history, and the various (often unusual) languages necessary to exploit nontraditional medical sources. At present, such people are extremely rare and in great demand.

The public must also reeducate itself. Laypeople, whether they are consumers of acupuncture, homeopathy, or maggot therapy, or innovators with a new potential cure for warts, multiple sclerosis, or Alzheimer's disease, have an obligation to understand the requirements of medical science. The more significant the claim of any alternative medicine, or the less well validated, the more skeptical the public must be and the more doubt the claimants must expect mainstream medical practitioners to express. Learning to address those doubts intelligently and scientifically will stimulate much progress. But the limits of that progress must also be understood. The fact is that the vast majority of promising drug leads pursued by pharmaceutical companies — as many as ninety-nine out of a hundred — never make it to market. Only one of three drugs that pharmaceutical and biotechnology companies bring before the FDA is approved for general use. We should not expect the winnowing process to be any easier for alternative medicines, especially in industrialized nations. Medical selection is never kind.

Nor should it be. The paramount issue on the long road from folk wisdom to the modern pharmacopoeia must always be the provision of the best possible medical care for each cultural environment. Folk wisdom must compete with the best that accepted medical practice can offer in any particular place, at any particular time. Honey, mud, and maggots, among many others, have competed and, so far, survived. Given the multitude of economic, social, and cultural environments the world over and the many innovations that have sprung from the reconsideration of diverse and discarded practices, we believe that other ancient and folk remedies will also yield medical understanding in the future. Indeed, mankind's medical achievement is already far broader than Western professional medicine has yet realized.

SELECTED BIBLIOGRAPHY

We examined more than a hundred books, over a thousand articles, and thousands of abstracts in preparing this book. When possible, we went back to primary sources to confirm or reconstruct the histories for ourselves. This bibliography therefore represents only a handful of critically important or easily available sources. Although the sources are listed by chapters, many of the articles and books contain material relevant to other topics, too.

INTRODUCTION. ANTIQUE MODERNITIES

Bynum, W. F., and R. Porter, eds. *Companion Encyclopedia of the History of Medicine,* 2 vols. London: Routledge, 1993.

Johnson, O. *Essay on West African Therapeutics.* New York: Trado-Medic Books, 1982.

Lyons, A. S., and J. Petrucelli. *Medicine: An Illustrated History.* New York: Abrams, 1978.

Majno, G. *The Healing Hand: Man and Wound in the Ancient World.* Cambridge, Mass.: Harvard University Press, 1975.

Peredo, M. G. *Medical Practices in Ancient America,* 2nd ed. Mexico City: Ediciones Euroamericanas, 1987.

Ray, P., H. N. Gupta, and N. Roy. *Suśruta Samhitā: A Scientific Synopsis.* New Delhi: Indian National Science Academy, 1980.

Sigerist, H. *A History of Medicine,* 2 vols. Oxford: Oxford University Press, 1951.

Schwab, C. W. *Cattle, Priests, and Progress in Medicine.* Minneapolis: University of Minnesota Press, 1978.

1. OLD WIVES' TALES AND THE CLINIC

Ackerknecht, E. H. *Therapeutics from the Primitives to the Twentieth Century.* New York: Macmillan, 1973.

Aikman, L. *Nature's Healing Arts: From Folk Medicine to Modern Drugs.* Washington: National Geographic Society, 1977.

Aronson, J. K. *An Account of the Foxglove and Its Medical Uses, 1785–1985.* London: Oxford University Press, 1985.

Colt, G. H. "See Me, Feel Me, Touch Me, Heal Me," *Life,* Sept. 1996, 34–50.

Eisner, R. "Botanists Ply Trade in Tropics, Seeking Plant-based Medicinals," *The Scientist* 5, no. 12 (1991): 1, 4–6.

Gordon, M. B. *Aesculapius Comes to the Colonies.* Ventnor, N.J., 1949.

Krantz, J. C. *Historical Medical Classics Involving New Drugs*. Baltimore: Williams and Wilkins, 1974.

Levine, I. E. *Conquerer of Smallpox: Dr. Edward Jenner.* New York: Julian Messner, 1960.

Mervis, J. "Ancient Remedy Performs New Tricks," *Science* 273 (1996): 578.

Ralston, J. "True Wives' Tales," *Allure*, May 1994: 142–49, 196–98.

Vogel, V. *American Indian Medicine*. Norman, Okla.: University of Oklahoma Press, 1970.

2. A FLYBLOWN IDEA

Baer, W. S. "Viable Antisepsis in Chronic Osteomyelitis," *Proceedings of the International Assembly of the Inter-State Postgraduate Medical Association of North America* 5 (1930): 370–72.

Blalock, D. "Grubby Little Secret: Maggots Are Neat at Fighting Infection," *Wall Street Journal*, 17 Jan. 1995: A1, A10.

Bunkis, J., S. Gherini, and R. Walton. "Maggot Therapy Revisited," *Western Journal of Medicine* 142 (1985): 554–56.

Dunbar, G. K. "Notes on the Ngemba Tribe of the Central Darling River, Western New South Wales," *Mankind* 3 (1944): 172–80.

Nolen, W. A. *The Making of a Surgeon*. New York: Random House, 1970.

Pechter, E., and R. Sherman. "Maggot Therapy: The Surgical Metamorphosis," *Plastic and Reconstructive Surgery* 72 (1983): 567–70.

Sherman, R. A., F. Wyle, and M. Vulpe. "Maggot Therapy for Treating Pressure Ulcers in Spinal Cord Injury Patients," *Journal of Spinal Cord Medicine* 18 (1995): 71–74.

Wilson, E. H., C. A. Doan, and D. F. Miller. "The Baer Maggot Treatment of Osteomyelitis," *Journal of the American Medical Association* 98 (1932): 1149–52.

Zimmer, C. "The Healing Power of Maggots," *Discover* 14, no. 8 (1993): 17.

3. SWEET TREAT(MENT)

Al Somal, N., K. E. Coley, P. C. Molan, and B. M. Hancock. "Susceptibility of *Helicobacter pylori* to the Antibacterial Activity of Manuka Honey," *Journal of the Royal Society of Medicine* 87 (1994): 9–12.

Cherife, J., L. Herszage, A. Joseph, and E. S. Kohn. "In Vitro Study of Bacterial Growth Inhibition in Concentrated Sugar Solutions: Microbiological Basis for the Use of Sugar in Treating Infected Wounds," *Antimicrobial Agents and Chemotherapy* 23 (1983): 766–73.

Davidson, J. R., and B. R. Ortiz de Montellano. "The Antibacterial Properties of an Aztec Wound Remedy," *Journal of Ethnopharmacology* 8 (1983): 149–61.

Jarvis, D. C. *Folk Medicine*. New York: Holt, Rinehart, and Winston, 1958.

Knutson, R. A., L. A. Merbitz, M. A. Creekmore, and H. G. Snipes. "Use of Sugar and Povidone-Iodine to Enhance Wound Healing: Five Years' Experience," *Southern Medical Journal* 74 (1981): 1329–35.

Postmes, T., A. E. van den Bogaard, and M. Hazen. "Honey for Wounds, Ulcers, and Skin Graft Preservation," *Lancet* 341 (1993): 756–57.

Singer, P. "Bioethics Where There Are Not Bioethicists." Video. Southfield, Mich.: Traditional Healing Productions, 1993.

Trouillet, J. L., J. Chastre, J. Y. Fagon, J. Pierre, Y. Domart, and C. Gibert. "Use of Granulated Sugar in Treatment of Open Mediastinitis after Cardiac Surgery," *Lancet* ii (1985): 180–84.

Zumla, A., and A. Lulat. "Honey — a Remedy Rediscovered," *Journal of the Royal Society of Medicine* 82 (1989): 384–85.

4. THE BABY IN THE BATH WATER

Conn, H. O. "Bath Is a Bath Is a Bath," *Hepatology* 6 (1986): 756–57.

Epstein, M. "Renal Effects of Head-out Water Immersion in Humans: A Fifteen-Year Update," *Journal of the American Physiological Society* 72 (1992): 563–621.

Fawthrop, F., N. Millar, A. E. A. Read, J. P. O'Hare, and C. F. M. Weston. "Combined Use of Water Immersion and Frusemide in Treatment of Resistant Ascites in Liver Cirrhosis," *Journal of the Royal Society of Medicine* 80 (1987): 776–77.

Heywood, A., H. A. Waldron, P. O'Hare, and P. A. Dieppe. "Effect of Immersion on Urinary Lead Excretion," *British Journal of Industrial Medicine* 43 (1986): 713–15.

Licht, S., ed. *Medical Hydrology*. Baltimore: Waverly Press, 1963.

Nicogossian, A. E., C. L. Huntoon, and S. L. Pool. *Space Physiology and Medicine*, 3rd ed. Philadelphia: Lea and Febiger, 1994.

O'Hare, J. P., A. Heywood, C. Summerhayes, G. Lunn, J. M. Evans, G. Walters, R. J. M. Corrall, and P. A. Dieppe. "Observations on the Effects of Immersion in Bath Spa Water," *British Medical Journal* 291 (1985): 1747–51.

Porter, R., ed. *The Medical History of Waters and Spas*. Medical History Suppl. no. 10. London: Wellcome Institute for the History of Medicine, 1990.

Thomson, W. A. R. *Spas That Heal*. London: Adam and Charles Black, 1978.

Waldron, H. A. "The Devonshire Colic," *Journal of the History of Medicine and Allied Sciences* 25, no. 4 (1970): 383–413.

5. GEOPHARMACY

Anell, B., and S. Lagercrantz. "Geophagical Customs," *Studia Ethnographical Upsaliensia* 17 (1958): vii–84.

Cooper, M. *Pica*. Springfield, Ill.: Charles C. Thomas, 1957.

Halsted, J. A. "Geophagia in Man: Its Nature and Nutritional Effects," *American Journal of Clinical Nutrition* 21 (1968): 1384–93.

Hunter, J. M. "Geophagy in Africa and in the United States," *Geographical Review* 63 (1973): 170–95.

Johns, T. "Detoxification Function of Geophagy and the Domestication of the Potato," *Journal of Chemical Ecology* 12 (1986): 635–46.

———. "Well-Grounded Diet: The Curious Practice of Eating Clay Is Rooted in Its Medicinal Value," *The Sciences*, Sept./Oct. 1991: 38–43.

Laufer, B. "Geophagy," *Field Museum of Natural History, Anthropological Series, Publication 280*, vol. 18, no. 2 (1930): 101–98.

Reid, R. M. "Cultural and Medical Perspectives on Geophagia," *Medical Anthropology* 13 (1992): 337–51.

Vermeer, D. E., and R. E. Farrell, Jr. "Nigerian Geophagical Clay: A Traditional Antidiarrheal Pharmaceutical," *Science* 227 (1985): 634–36.

Vermeer, D. E., and D. A. Frate. "Geophagia in Rural Mississippi: Environmental and Cultural Contexts and Nutritional Implications," *American Journal of Clinical Nutrition* 32 (1979): 2129–35.

6. A BLOODY GOOD REMEDY

Burch, G. E., and N. P. DePasquale. "Phlebotomy: Use in Patients with Erythrocytosis and Ischemic Heart Disease," *Archives of Internal Medicine* 111 (1963): 687–95.

Carpenter, C. C. "The Erratic Evolution of Cholera Therapy: From Folklore to Science," *Clinical Therapeutic* 12, suppl. A (1990): 22–27.

Casale, G., M. Bignamini, and P. de Nicola. "Does Blood Donation Prolong Life Expectancy?" *Vox Sanguinus* 45 (1983): 398–99.

Crosby, W. "A History of Phlebotomy Therapy for Hemochromatosis," *American Journal of the Medical Sciences* 301 (1991): 28–31.

Kasting, N. "A Rationale for Centuries of Therapeutic Bloodletting: Antipyretic Therapy for Febrile Diseases," *Perspectives in Biology and Medicine* 33 (1990): 509–16.

Kluger, M. J. "The History of Bloodletting," *Natural History* 87, Nov. 1978: 78–83.

"Phlebotomy: An Ancient Procedure Turning Modern?" *Journal of the American Medical Association* 183 (1963): 147–48.

Sullivan, J. L. "The Iron Paradigm of Ischemic Heart Disease," *American Heart Journal* 117 (1989): 1177–88.

———. "Blood Donation May Be Good for the Donor: Iron, Heart Disease, and Donor Recruitment," *Vox Sanguinus* 61 (1991): 161–64.

7. HIRUDO THE HERO

Davis, A., and T. Appel. *Bloodletting Instruments in the National Museum of History and Technology.* Washington: Smithsonian Institution Press, 1979.

Derganc, M., and F. Zdravic. "Venous Congestion of Flaps Treated by Application of Leeches," *British Journal of Plastic Surgery* 13 (1960): 187–92.

Fackelmann, K. A. "Bloodsuckers Reconsidered: Leech Saliva Inspires a Medical Quest," *Science News* 139 (1991): 172–73.

Fields, W. S. "The History of Leeching and Hirudin," *Haemostasis* 21, suppl. 1 (1991): 3–10.

Kraemer, B. A., K. E. Korber, T. I. Aquino, and A. Engleman. "Use of Leeches in Plastic and Reconstructive Surgery: A Review," *Journal of Reconstructive Microsurgery* 4 (1988): 381–85.

Lent, C. "New Medical and Scientific Uses of the Leech," *Nature* 323 (1986): 494.

Rao, P., F. B. Bailie, and B. N. Bailey. "Leechmania in Microsurgery," *The Practitioner* 229 (1985): 901–5.
Sawyer, R. T. "Why We Need to Save the Medicinal Leech," *Oryx* 16 (1981): 165–68.
———. *Leech Biology and Behaviour,* 2 vols. Oxford: Clarendon Press, 1986.

8. LAUDABLE PUS

Colebrook, L. *Almroth Wright: Provocative Doctor and Thinker.* London: Heinemann, 1954.
Cope, Z. "The Treatment of Wounds Through the Ages," *Medical History* 2 (1958): 163–73.
Edwards, P. D. *Alexis Carrel: Visionary Surgeon.* Springfield, Ill.: Charles C. Thomas, 1974.
Herriot, J. *James Herriot's Dog Stories* (new introduction and notes). New York: St. Martin's Press, 1987.
Higgs, S. L., J. Trueta, and R. Brooke. "Discussion of the Closed Plaster Treatment of Wounds in the Light of Recent Experience," *Proceedings of the Royal Society of Medicine* 34 (1941): 218–21.
Hunt, T. K., and B. Halliday. "Inflammation in Wounds: From 'Laudable Pus' to Primary Repair and Beyond." In *Wound Healing and Wound Infection, Theory and Surgical Practice,* ed. T. K. Hunt. New York: Appleton-Century-Crofts, 1980.
Levenson, S. M., D. Kan-Gruber, C. Gruber, J. Molnar, and E. Seifter. "Wound Healing Accelerated by *Staphylococcus aureus,*" *Archives of Surgery* 118 (1983): 310–20.
Orr, H. W. "Treatment of Fractures by Means of Skeletal Devices: Fixation in Plaster-of-Paris Casts," *Journal of the American Medical Association* 98 (1932): 947–51.
Rous, P. "The Activation of Skin Grafts," *Journal of Experimental Medicine* 83 (1946): 383–400.
Trueta, J. *Treatment of War Wounds and Fractures.* New York: Paul B. Hoeber, 1940.

9. LICKING INFECTION

Bodner, L., A. Knyszynski, S. Adler-Kunin, and D. Danon. "The Effect of Selective Desalivation on Wound Healing in Mice," *Experimental Gerontology* 26 (1991): 357–63.
Hart, B. L., and K. L. Powell. "Antibacterial Properties of Saliva: Role in Maternal Periparturient Grooming and in Licking Wounds," *Physiology of Behavior* 48 (1990): 383–86.
Levi-Montalcini, R. *In Praise of Imperfection: My Life and Work.* New York: Basic Books, 1988.
Levine, M. J. "Development of Artificial Salivas," *Critical Reviews of Oral Biology and Medicine* 4 (1993): 279–86.
Malamud, D., and H. M. Friedman. "HIV in the Oral Cavity: Virus, Viral Inhibi-

263

tory Activity, and Antiviral Antibodies: A Review," *Critical Reviews of Oral Biology and Medicine* 4 (1993): 461–66.

Mandel, I. D. "The Functions of Saliva," *Journal of Dental Research* 66, special no. (1987): 623–27.

Meyer-Ingold, M. "Wound Therapy: Growth Factors as Agents to Promote Healing," *Trends in Biotechnology* 11 (1993): 387–92.

Root-Bernstein, R. S. *Discovering*. Cambridge, Mass.: Harvard University Press, 1989.

Sherertz, E. F. "Why Sadie Licks Her Wounds," *Archives of Dermatology* 124 (1988): 1499–1500.

Verrier, L. "Dog Licks Man," *Lancet* i (1970): 615.

10. UROTHERAPY

Armstrong, J. W. *The Water of Life*, 2nd ed. London: True Health Publishing, 1944.

Chuinard, E. G. *Only One Man Died: The Medical Aspects of the Lewis and Clark Expedition*. Glendale, Calif.: Arthur H. Clark, 1979.

Ortiz de Montellano, B. R. "Aztec Sources of Some Mexican Folk Medicine." In *Folk Medicine: The Art and the Science*, ed. R. P. Steiner. Washington: American Chemical Society, 1986.

Gelfand, M., S. Mavi, R. B. Drummond, and B. Ndemera. *The Traditional Medical Practitioner in Zimbabwe: His Principles of Practice and Pharmacopoeia*. Gweru, Zimbabwe: Mambo Press, 1985.

Heath, P. "Amoroli: The Ancient Practice of Urine Therapy," *Continuum Magazine*, no. 4 (June/July 1993): 3.

Herman, J. R. "Autourotherapy: The Water of Life," *New York State Journal of Medicine* 80 (1980): 1149–54.

Mills, M. H., and T. A. Faunce. "Melatonin Supplementation from Early Morning Auto-Urine Drinking," *Medical Hypotheses* 36 (1991): 195–99.

Mueller, R. L., and S. Scheidt. "History of Drugs for Thrombotic Disease: Discovery, Development, and Directions for the Future," *Circulation* 89 (1994): 432–49.

Needham, J., and G.-D. Lu. "Sex Hormones in the Middle Ages," *Endeavor* 27 (1968): 130–32.

Walburn, J. N., J. M. Pergam, S. H. Perry, and J. Jensen. "Black Child Care Practices in the Midwest," *Pediatrics* 82 (1988): 789–90.

11. FULL CIRCLE

Cook, L. S., L. A. Koutsky, and K. K. Holmes. "Circumcision and Sexually Transmitted Diseases," *American Journal of Public Health* 84 (1994): 197–201.

Ewings, P., and C. Bowie. "A Case-Control Study of Cancer of the Prostate in Somerset and East Devon," *British Journal of Cancer* 74 (1996): 661–66.

Gollaher, D. L. "From Ritual to Science: The Medical Transformation of Circumcision in America," *Journal of Social History*, Fall 1994: 5–35.

Grossman, E.A., and N. A. Posner. "The Circumcision Controversy: An Update," *Obstetrics Gynecology Annual* 13 (1984): 181–95.

James, T. "Philo on Circumcision," *South African Medical Journal,* 21 Aug. 1976: 1409–12.

Moses, S., F. A. Plummer, J. E. Bradley, J. O. Ndinya-Achola, N. J. Nagelkerke, and A. R. Ronald. "The Association between Lack of Male Circumcision and Risk of HIV Infection: A Review of the Epidemiological Data," *Sexually Transmitted Diseases* 21 (1994): 201–10.

Remondino, P. C. *History of Circumcision.* Philadelphia: Davis, 1900.

Ross, R. K., H. Shimizu, A. Paganini-Hill, G. Honda, and B. E. Henderson. "Case-Control Studies of Prostate Cancer in Blacks and Whites in Southern California," *Journal of the National Cancer Institute* 78 (1987): 869–74.

Schoen, E. J. "Neonatal Circumcision and Penile Cancer: Evidence That Circumcision Is Protective Is Overwhelming," *British Medical Journal* 313 (1996): 46.

Wiswell, T. E., and W. E. Hachey. "Urinary Tract Infections and the Uncircumcised State: An Update," *Clinical Pediatrics* 32 (1993): 130–34.

12. A CONTRACEPTIVE MISCONCEPTION

Farnsworth, N. R., A. S. Bingel, G. A. Cordell, F. A. Crane, and H. H. S. Fong. "Potential Value of Plants as Sources of New Antifertility Agents: II," *Journal of Pharmaceutical Sciences* 64 (1975): 717–54.

Himes, N. E. *Medical History of Contraception.* Baltimore: Williams and Wilkins, 1936.

Jöchle, W. "Menses-Inducing Drugs: Their Role in Antique, Medieval and Renaissance Gynecology and Birth Control," *Contraception* 10 (1974): 425–39.

Keown, K. K., Jr. "Historical Perspectives on Intravaginal Contraceptive Sponges," *Contraception* 16 (1977): 1–10.

Kong, Y. C., J.-X. Xei, and P. P.-H. But. "Fertility Regulating Agents from Traditional Chinese Medicines," *Journal of Ethnopharmacology* 15 (1986): 1–44.

McClaren, A. *A History of Contraception from Antiquity to the Present Day.* Cambridge, Mass.: Basil Blackwell, 1990.

Riddle, J. M. *Contraception and Abortion from the Ancient World to the Renaissance.* Cambridge, Mass.: Harvard University Press, 1992.

Riddle, J. M., and J. W. Estes. "Oral Contraceptives in Ancient and Medieval Times," *American Scientist* 80 (1992): 226–33.

Wheeler, D. L. "A Fresh Direction for Birth Control," *Chronicle of Higher Education* 42, no. 39 (1996): A10.

Youssef, H. "The History of the Condom," *Journal of the Royal Society of Medicine* 86 (1993): 226–28.

13. UNDER WRAPS

Allen, O. E. "Sticky Business," *Invention & Technology* 10, no. 3 (1995): 48–52.

Bloom, H. "'Cellophane' Dressing for Second-Degree Burns," *Lancet,* no. 2 (Nov. 3, 1945): 559.

Chistyakov, N. L. "The Use of Cellophane in the Treatment of Wounds" (in Russian), *Khirurgiya* 7 (1944): 32–37; Eng. trans., *American Review of Soviet Medicine* 3 (1946): 490–93.

Cuzzell, J. Z., and N. A. Stotts. "Wound Care: Trial and Error Leads to Knowledge," *American Journal of Nursing* (Oct. 1990): 53–63.

Elder, A. V. "Cellophane as a Surgical Dressing," *Journal of the Royal Navy Medical Service* 24 (1938): 154–55.

Ellis, M. "Transparent Wrapping Material for Dressing Open Wounds and Ulcers," *British Medical Journal,* June 5, 1943: 697.

Farr, J. "'Cellophane' for the Treatment of Burns," *British Medical Journal,* June 3, 1944: 749–50.

Houghton, R. H., et al. "Bacteriostasis of *Staphylococcus aureus* by a Volatile Component of 'Scotch' Brand Cellulose Adhesive Tape," *Nature* 201 (1964): 1346–47.

Howes, E. L. "Cellophane as a Wound Dressing," *Surgery* 6 (1939): 426–27.

Kimbrough, J. W. "New Cellophane Dressing," *United States Naval Medical Bulletin* 40 (1942): 432–35.

14. UNNATURAL SELECTION

Alland, A., Jr. *Adaptation in Cultural Evolution: An Approach to Medical Anthropology.* New York: Columbia University Press, 1970.

Chagnon, N. A., and W. Irons, eds. *Evolutionary Biology and Human Social Behavior.* New York: Columbia University Press, 1979.

Dobzhansky, T., and E. Boesiger. *Human Culture: A Moment in Evolution.* New York: Columbia University Press, 1983.

Epstein, M., ed. *The Kidney in Liver Disease,* 3rd ed. Baltimore: Williams and Wilkins, 1988.

Leake, C. D. *The Old Egyptian Medical Papyri.* Lawrence, Kans.: University of Kansas Press, 1952.

McAuliffe, K. "What the Witch Doctor Knew," *Good Housekeeping/Living Well,* Apr. 1992: 156–58.

———. "Continuum: Shaman Pharmaceuticals," *Omni* 15 (July 1993): 27.

Roach, M. "Secrets of the Shamans," *Discover* 14, no. 11 (Nov. 1993): 58–65.

Root-Bernstein, R. S. "Hindsight on Medicine," *The Sciences,* Mar.–Apr., 1991: 10–12.

15. APING THE APES

Cowen, R. "Medicine on the Wild Side," *Science News* 138 (1990): 280–82.

Fossey, D. *Gorillas in the Mist.* Boston: Houghton Mifflin, 1983.

Gibbons, A. "Plants of the Apes," *Science* 255 (1992): 921.

Goodall, J. *The Chimpanzees of Gombe: Patterns of Behavior.* Cambridge, Mass.: Belknap Press of Harvard University Press, 1986.

Morris, D. *The Naked Ape.* London: Jonathan Cape, 1967.

———. *Animal Watching.* New York: Crown Books, 1990.

Newton, P., and T. Nishida. "Possible Buccal Administration of Herbal Drugs by Wild Chimpanzees *(Pan troglodytes)*," *Animal Behavior* 39 (1991): 799–800.

Nishida, T., and M. Nakamura. "Chimpanzee Tool Use to Clear a Blocked Nasal Passage," *Folia Primatologia* 61 (1993): 218–20.

Ritchie, B. G., and D. M. Fragaszy. "Capuchin Monkey *(Cebus apella)* Grooms Her Infant's Wound with Tools," *American Journal of Primatology* 16 (1988): 345–48.

Rodriguez, E., M. Aregullin, T. Nishida, S. Uehara, R. Wrangham, et al. "Thiarubrine A, a Bioactive Constituent of *Aspilia* (Asteraceae) Consumed by Wild Chimpanzees," *Experientia* 41 (1985): 419–20.

Westergaard, G., and D. M. Fragaszy. "Self-Treatment of Wounds by a Capuchin Monkey *(Cebus apella)*," *Human Evolution* 2 (1987): 557–62.

16. INDIGENOUS HEALING

Bohannan, L. "Shakespeare in the Bush." In *Ants, Indians and Little Dinosaurs*, ed. A. Ternes. New York: Charles Scribner's Sons, 1975.

Bulatao, R. A., J. A. Palmore, and S. E. Ward, eds. *Choosing a Contraceptive: Method Choice in Asia and the United States*. San Francisco: Westview Press, 1989.

Carpio, B. A., and B. Majumdar. "Experiential Learning: An Approach to Transcultural Education for Nursing," *Journal of Transcultural Nursing* 4 (1993): 4–11.

Giger, J. N., R. E. Davidhizar, and G. Turner. "Black American Folk Medicine Health Care Beliefs: Implications for Nursing Plans of Care," *ABNF Journal* 3, no. 2 (1992): 42–46.

Harwood, A., ed. *Ethnicity and Medical Care*. Cambridge, Mass.: Harvard University Press, 1981.

Lum, C. K., and S. G. Korenman. "Cultural-Sensitivity Training in U.S. Medical Schools," *Academic Medicine* 69 (1994): 239–41.

MacCormack, C. P. "Primary Health Care in Sierra Leone," *Social Science Medicine* 19, no. 3 (1984): 199–208.

Schweiger, A., and A. Parducci. "Nocebo: The Psychologic Induction of Pain," *Pavlov Journal of Biological Science* 16 (1981): 140–43.

Trotter, R. T., II. "Folk Remedies as Indicators of Common Illnesses: Examples from the United States–Mexico Border," *Journal of Ethnopharmacology* 4 (1981): 207–21.

Werner, D., C. Thuman, and J. Maxwell. *Where There Is No Doctor: A Village Health Care Handbook*. Palo Alto: Hesperian Foundation, 1992.

17. CRACKPOTS AND PANACEAS

Brown, C. "The Experiments of Dr. Oz," *New York Times Magazine*, 30 July, 1995: 21–23.

Carr, A. "Bitten by a Fer-de-Lance." In *Ants, Indians and Little Dinosaurs*, ed. A. Ternes. New York: Charles Scribner's Sons, 1975.

Cohen, M., et al. *Melatonin: From Contraception to Breast Cancer Prevention*. Potomac, Md.: Sheba Press, 1995.

Food and Drug Administration. "The Top Ten Health Care Frauds," *FDA Consumer,* Feb. 1990: 34–36.

Glasscheib, H. S. *The March of Medicine: Aberrations and Triumphs of the Healing Art.* London: Macdonald, 1961.

Hamburg, J. "Quack Cures and Health Frauds," *Family Circle,* 27 Apr., 1993: 136–38.

Michelmore, P. "Beware the Health Hucksters," *Reader's Digest,* Jan. 1989: 114–18.

Soffer, A. "Chihuahuas and Laetrile, Chelation Therapy, and Honey from Boulder, Colo.," *Archives of Internal Medicine* 136 (1976): 865–66.

Trachtman, P. "NIH Looks at the Implausible and the Inexplicable," *Smithsonian,* Sept. 1994: 110–21.

CONCLUSION: FROM FOLK WISDOM TO PHARMACOPOEIA

Caulfield, C. R., and B. Goldberg. *The Anarchist AIDS Medical Formulary: A Guide to Guerilla Immunology.* Berkeley: North Atlantic Books, 1993.

Cimons M. "New Life for Old Remedies," *Los Angeles Times,* 1 Jan. 1996: A1, A16.

DiMasi, J., H. Grabowski, L. Lasagna, and R. Hansen. "The Cost of Innovation in the Pharmaceutical Industry," *Journal of Health Economics* 10 (1990): 107–20.

Mack, A. "Biotechnology Turns to Ancient Remedies in Quest for Sources of New Therapies," *The Scientist,* 6 Jan. 1997: 1, 8–9.

Nowak, R. "Chronobiologists Out of Sync over Light Therapy Patents," *Science* 263 (1994): 1217–18.

Root-Bernstein, R. S. "The Development and Dissemination of Non-Patentable Therapies (NPTs)," *Perspectives in Biology and Medicine* 39 (1995): 110–17.

Stricker, R. B., et al. "Pilot Study of Topical Dinitrochlorobenzene (DNCB) in HIV Infection," *Immunology Letters* 36 (1993): 1–6.

Witte, M. H., A. Kerwin, C. L. Witte, and A. Scadron. "A Curriculum on Medical Ignorance," *Medical Education* 23 (1989): 24–29.

INDEX